"The authors set out to give Playback Theatre a theoretical and clinical base for use in Group Psychotherapy, and they succeed! Drawing on the rich tradition of Non-Scripted Theatre and integrating it with psychodynamic psychotherapy, this book is an important, groundbreaking contribution to the field, rich in clinical perspectives. I highly recommend it!"

David Read Johnson, Ph.D., *RDT-BCT, director,*
Institute of Developmental Transformations. Co-editor,
Current Approaches in Drama Therapy, *Charles C*
Thomas, 2020

"A thoughtful, sensitive guided tour of a method of group psychotherapy integrating psychoanalytic and psychodramatic approaches. Well grounded in theory, the stories are much more than standard clinical case material. Engaging and clearly written, the authors bring the process to life. Creative clinicians and the interested public can participate."

Robert W Siroka, Ph.D., *founder,*
The Sociometric Institute, NYC

"This book represents a real gem. It combines the systematic use of playback theatre for therapeutic realms with a group analytic perspective. It introduces moreover Jungian concepts to amplify its theoretical and practical scope. Readers from both active and reflective group approaches will surely benefit from its stimulating ideas."

Dr. Jorge Burmeister, *former president, IAGP*

"This book is a bridge between Playback Theatre and psychoanalytic group psychotherapy. Each chapter weaves together philosophical ideas from theatre, psychoanalysis, psychodrama, and drama therapy with carefully chosen examples that illuminate important clinical considerations. It is an invitation to therapists to develop imaginative, playful capacities in the context of group work and explore applications in a variety of contexts."

Nisha Sajnani, Ph.D., *RDT-BCT, director, NYU*
Program in Drama Therapy

"A warm welcome for this original and valuable book. Psychotherapeutic Playback Theatre is a new, inventive approach that that has much potential at a time of widespread emotional stress. I enjoyed the playful approach of the method, clearly and convincingly described. Yet, the book reveals an erudition and scholarship that make it a serious contribution to the field. The method, while having light, playful aspects, is capable of reaching emotional depth in individuals and groups. It is a tribute to the authors that I felt a distinct urge to participate in a playback therapy group myself! I suspect

T0372863

other readers may feel the same. In the meantime, reading the book is an excellent preparation."

Morris Nitsun, *psychologist, psychotherapist, training group analyst, Institute of Group Analysis, London. Author of* The Anti-group *and* The Group as an object of Desire. *Practising, exhibiting artist*

"This book is much needed in the group therapy field. It is the first book ever written about psychotherapeutic playback theatre and as such, it illuminates an important and neglected area in group therapy modalities... Playback theatre can be a powerful way to see others "act your problems" and create different endings that help you heal. Ronen Kowalsky, Nir Raz and Shoshi Keisari are to be commended for their achievement in writing and publishing this book."

Haim Weinberg, *clinical psychologist, group analyst & group psychotherapist. Former president of the Northern California Group Therapy Society. Writer of numerous books and articles about group therapy*

"...This book is creating an interwove of theories and models that were individually presented such as Psychodrama, Dramatherapy and Analytic group work (and more) into a new set of insights, methods and practices creating a novel and creative structure both for practitioners and scholars to look into the healing potential of Psychotherapeutic Playback Theater. The book, full of case examples and references is a great resource for students of drama, theater, Arts therapists, and other psychotherapists interested in action therapies. In my view this book presents the power of traditional inter-being process of healing using variety of art form methods with the postmodern concepts of 'therapy'."

Mooli Lahad, Ph.D., *founder of Dramatherapy in Israel. Full Professor of Psychology and Dramatherapy, Tel Hai College. Founder and president of the Community Stress Prevention Center, Israel*

An Introduction to Psychotherapeutic Playback Theater: Hall of Mirrors on Stage by Ronen Kowalsky, Nir Raz and Shoshi Keisari gives an interesting account of a form of group psychotherapy developed in Israel that combines theatrical and psychoanalytic traditions. In the background are J. L. Moreno's psychodrama and the Playback Theater of J. Fox. These theatrical traditions are here skillfully merged with psychoanalytic ideas from W. Bion, such as the container and contained, as well as S. H. Foulkes's notion of resonance. The authors offer numerous examples of the method throughout. There are also interesting chapters on an expanded notion of dramatic reality (by Susana Pendzik) and on the influence of French Surre-alism on working with dreamlike states. I would recommend this book to group therapists with an interest in cross-fertilization of techniques from different schools and traditions. This manages to be both an exciting and scholarly book."

Dominick Grundy, Ph.D., *Fellow, American Group Psychotherapy Association, Former editor, International Journal of Group Psychotherapy*

"Here is something new – a sound and fascinating integration of playback theatre and analytic group therapy. Drawing from group analysis, object relations psychoanalysis, psychodrama, creative arts therapy, theatre, and surrealism, *An Introduction to Psychotherapeutic Playback Theater: Hall of Mirrors on Stage* stands on the pillars of Moreno, Fox, Salas, Winnicott, and Bion. Its authors open a door to an emerging field, a vast space for exploring the psyche and the social-collective dimension of experience by combining therapeutic groups and theatre techniques. Recalling a Bion quote, 'Beauty can hold the most difficult truth and make it easier to digest,' the authors and their clinical illustrations prove that with the theatrical aesthetic as con-tainer, the individual story becomes an illuminating collective experience, by retelling, expanding and revealing deeper layers during a deep, emotional and direct encounter between the individual and the group. This book will be of great interest to group therapists, counsellors, facilitators, mediators, and actors who want to deepen their understanding of the human condition – and intervene effectively using the authors' unique method of psychothera-peutic playback theatre."

Jill Savege Scharff, MD, *FABP, FTCL, LGSM; Co-founder, International Psychotherapy Institute. Author of* Doctor in the House Seat: Psychoanalytic Perspectives on Theatre *(2013)*

"...This is the first book of its kind to bring playback as a group psychotherapy therapy process. You can find in these wonderful texts a whole theoretical and practical set based on tools from the field of Playback Theater, im-provisation, theater games, group dynamic and psychoanalytic theories. Creative arts Therapists, psychodrama, drama therapists, Playback theater practitioners with a therapeutic orientation, and anyone involved in group work, may find in this book an inexhaustible source of knowledge, guid-ance, support and inspiration."

Aviva Apel Rosenthal, *theater director, creative arts therapist. Former president of IPT, CPT – leadership teacher and PB advance skills trainer, founder and director of "Play Life" PBT*

An Introduction to Psychotherapeutic Playback Theater

An Introduction to Psychotherapeutic Playback Theater is a comprehensive book presenting Psychotherapeutic Playback Theater as a unique form of group psychotherapy.

This pioneering book is the first of its kind, examining this new approach, the theory behind it, and the numerous considerations and diverse possibilities involved in using the technique to promote a significant reflective process among participants. Informed by years of Psychotherapeutic Playback Theater practice and research, the authors detail a collective-creative method that allows for the creation of a therapeutic experience centered on feelings of belonging, acceptance, visibility and liberation. It is presented to the reader as a path toward their development and growth as a conductor working in this newly evolving field of group therapy.

The book will be of great interest to dramatherapy students, trainees and professionals, and group therapists who wish to reflect upon their practice through the mirror of Psychotherapeutic Playback Theater as well as facilitators and actors working with Playback Theater or other improvised genres.

Ronen Kowalsky, M.A., is a supervising clinical psychologist, co-founder and head of the Israeli Institute of Psychotherapeutic Playback Theater and member of the Israeli Institute of Group Analysis. He is faculty and supervisor at the Winnicott Center and the Academic College of Society and Art.

Nir Raz is an international Playback Theater trainer, writer and stage artist, and co-founder and head of the Israeli Institute of Psychotherapeutic Playback Theater. He teaches at the Schneider Clown-care Academy, and is a medical clown and hydrotherapist.

Shoshi Keisari, Ph.D., is a drama therapist and scholar in the field of drama therapy and clinical gerontology. She is a lecturer and a researcher at the School of Creative Arts Therapies and the Emilie Sagol Creative Arts Therapies Research Center at the university of Haifa, Israel.

Susana Pendzik, Ph.D., RDT, former head of the Drama Therapy M.A. program at Tel-Hai College, Israel, and lecturer at the Theatre Studies Department of the Hebrew University of Jerusalem, the Dramatherapy Swiss Institute and other academic institutions worldwide.

The New International Library of Group Analysis (NILGA)
Series Editor: Earl Hopper

Drawing on the seminal ideas of British, European and American group analysts, psychoanalysts, social psychologists and social scientists, the books in this series focus on the study of small and large groups, organisations and other social systems, and on the study of the transpersonal and transgenerational sociality of human nature. NILGA books will be required reading for the members of professional organisations in the field of group analysis, psychoanalysis, and related social sciences. They will be indispensable for the "formation" of students of psychotherapy, whether they are mainly interested in clinical work with patients or in consultancy to teams and organisational clients within the private and public sectors.

Recent titles in the series include:

Addressing Challenging Moments in Psychotherapy
Clinical Wisdom for Working with Individuals, Groups and Couples
Edited by Jerome S. Gans

Psychoanalysis, Group Analysis, and Beyond
Towards a New Paradigm of the Human Being
Juan Tubert-Oklander and Reyna Hernández-Tubert

An Introduction to Psychotherapeutic Playback Theater
Hall of Mirrors on Stage
Ronen Kowalsky, Nir Raz and Shoshi Keisari with Susana Pendzik

Psycho-social Explorations of Trauma, Exclusion and Violence
Un-housed Minds and Inhospitable Environments
Christopher Scanlon and John Adlam

For more information about this series, please visit: https://www.routledge.com/Routledge-Studies-in-Genocide-and-Crimes-against-Humanity/book-series/RSGCH

An Introduction to Psychotherapeutic Playback Theater

Hall of Mirrors on Stage

Ronen Kowalsky, Nir Raz and
Shoshi Keisari with Susana Pendzik

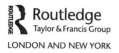

Routledge
Taylor & Francis Group

LONDON AND NEW YORK

Cover art by Anna Ponomariova

First published 2022
by Routledge
4 Park Square, Milton Park, Abingdon, Oxon OX14 4RN

and by Routledge
605 Third Avenue, New York, NY 10158

Routledge is an imprint of the Taylor & Francis Group, an informa business

British Library Cataloguing-in-Publication Data
A catalogue record for this book is available from the British Library

Library of Congress Cataloging-in-Publication Data
Names: Kowalsky, Ronen, author. | Raz, Nir, author. | Keisari, Shoshi,
author. | Pendzik, Susana, other.
Title: An introduction to psychotherapeutic playback theater: hall of
mirrors on stage / Ronen Kowalsky, Nir Raz and Shoshi Keisari with
Susana Pendzik.
Description: Milton Park, Abingdon, Oxon; New York, NY: Routledge,
2022. |
Series: The new international library of group analysis | Includes
bibliographical references and index. | Identifiers: LCCN 2021040373
(print) | LCCN 2021040374 (ebook) | ISBN 9780367766306 (hardback)
| ISBN 9780367766290 (paperback) | ISBN 9781003167822 (ebook)
Subjects: LCSH: Drama—Therapeutic use. | Group psychotherapy.
Classification: LCC RC489.P7 K69 2022 (print) | LCC RC489.P7
(ebook) | DDC 616.89/1523—dc23
LC record available at https://lccn.loc.gov/2021040373
LC ebook record available at https://lccn.loc.gov/2021040374

ISBN: 9780367766306 (hbk)
ISBN: 9780367766290 (pbk)
ISBN: 9781003167822 (ebk)

DOI: 10.4324/9781003167822

Typeset in Times New Roman
by codeMantra

Translated by Amir Atsmon
Illustrations by Anna Ponomariova

Originally published in Hebrew in 2019 as:
"Heichal Hamarot al Habama: Psychoterapia Beteatron
Playback"
by The Emily Sagol Arts Therapy Research Center,
Haifa University.

Contents

Acknowledgments

First and foremost, we would like to thank the dear people at Routledge Publishing House, who showed faith in the novel ideas presented in this book and accompanied us in preparing its English version: Dr. Earl Hopper, who made this version a reality with his endless and contagious enthusiasm and curiosity and whose every remark deepened and expanded our thinking; Alexis O'Brian and Alec Slavin, who believed in this book and saw it through to publication.

We would like to thank Jo Salas and Jonathan Fox, who created the marvelous form of theater that is the inspiration and the foundation of the psychotherapeutic method presented in this book. We would like to thank our friends in the international and Israeli Playback Theater communities, whose evolving work since the 1970s served as the habitat where our ideas could grow.

We are grateful to our many friends who make up the human tapestry of Psychotherapeutic Playback Theater. We would like to extend our heartfelt thanks to the staff of the Institute of Psychotherapeutic Playback Theater, who played a big part in developing the ideas presented in this book – Galila Oren, Dr. Avi Bauman, Dr. Yael Doron and Eli Hacham. We especially thank Pazit Ilan Berkowitz, who has been nurturing and encouraging our ideas from the very beginning; and Professor Susana Pendzik, who added and contributed a chapter to this book, presenting her unique way of thinking. We are also grateful to Aviva Apel and Nili Lubrani Rolnik, two leading figures of Playback Theater in Israel and worldwide, whom we were fortunate to welcome to our institute's staff. We have benefitted greatly from each and every step in our ongoing dialogue with them.

Special thanks also go to Yehuda Bergman, for introducing the field of Playback Theater to Ronen and giving him the opportunity to teach Playback Theater in different drama therapy departments. We also thank Prof. Mooli Lahad for opening the door to this world wide open. We are very glad that he joined the institute right from its very beginning.

We thank Yoram Chen and Einat Mishal for introducing Nir to the world of Playback Theater; we are grateful to Pazit Ilan Berkowitz and the "Mar'ot" Ensemble for their partnership, friendship, creativity and development.

We are grateful to Prof. Yuval Palgi, Prof. Anat Gesser-Edelsberg and Dr. Danny Yaniv for their guidance of Shoshi's research on Playback Theater and the Third Age. This primary encounter of the aging population with Psychotherapeutic Playback Theater deepened our understanding and validated the qualities of the process.

Many thanks to Prof. Rachel Lev-Wiesel, Danielle Friedlander and the Emili Sagol Creative Arts Therapies Research Center at the University of Haifa's Faculty of Social Welfare and Health Sciences, for believing in us and encouraging us to publish the original Hebrew version of this book. We also thank Dr. Hod Orkivi for the open door and for believing in us and our approach.

We would also like to thank the energetic team that accompanied us throughout the various stages of writing this book, for bringing it to its current level – our scientific editor, Dr. Yehudit Rivko; and our illustrator, Anna Ponomeriova. A special thank you goes to our translator – Amir Atsmon – whose determined search for the right words sharpened our ideas to the extent that we eventually published a revised Hebrew edition based on the changes made in the English translation.

We would like to thank our students at the Institute: experienced therapists who, over a period of two years, spent one day each week deepening and broadening their understanding of this new field. Some of them – including a co-author of this book – have already become supervisors and teachers at the Institute. Special thanks go to Ayelet Mosenzon and Lilach Weiner for transcribing our lectures, which were used as the raw material for this book. We also thank all the different people who, over the years, had been members of the "Incubator" Psychotherapeutic Playback Theater group, in which many of the ideas discussed in this book were developed.

We thank the patients in our groups and those of our students and graduates, in psychiatric wards and clinics in both hospital and community settings; in centers for holocaust survivors and centers for those coping with mental difficulties; in empowerment groups for rehabilitated alcohol and drug addicts, in community-based settings for psychiatric care, schools and various settings for the aging population. This new field of therapy belongs to you just as much as it does to us.

And, finally, we extend our especially warm thanks to our beloved families, for their patience and generous support.

Foreword

Ronen Kowalsky, Nir Raz and Shoshi Keisari

Beyond smell, touch and taste the survival and development of each and all of us depends on our ability and willingness to see and to hear. This configuration of senses is the crucible of knowing, but ultimately what is known, both generally and specifically, is also function of what there is to be known. Creation is always co-creation, especially with respect to social and psychic facts and processes. Axiomatic to Group Analysis, the recognition and appreciation of this relational insight involves a tremendous shock to our fantasies and phantasies of omnipotence and omniscience. Our need to regulate this insult to our narcissism is most probably at the root of our religious and political impulses, involving connection and re-connection, and attempting to make sense of the experience of helplessness.

The expression of these Ur-themes during the early 20th century has of course been traced to the work of several European sociologists, psychoanalysts and nascent group and community therapists, including psychodramatists. However, S. H. Foulkes himself acknowledged what he called the "germinal influence" of Pirandello's (1995) *Six Characters in Search of an Author* and Gorki's (2008) *The Lower Depths.* Like the rest of us, he was also influenced by his "reading" of the great Greek tragedies, especially "Oedipus Tyrannus." He was especially interested in the way that group process was portrayed in various plays, e.g., those of Chekhov. From time to time these influences have been acknowledged and discussed, for example by Thompson (1983) and Roth (2014). More recently, Wilke (2021) has referred to the neglected role and functions of the "chorus," who unconsciously bears witness to the relations between protagonists and antagonists, which is analogous to the relations among observers, perpetrators and victims. We are so often in denial of the dynamics of our own internal worlds, as we see and hear so much violence and terrorism in our external worlds.

I remember that during the 1960s, which for the Institute of Group Analysis (IGA) (London) was a kind of "dream time," I was asked to teach a seminar on sociological ideas that might be important in clinical group analysis. I readily and enthusiastically accepted this somewhat creative invitation. However, to the surprise of the Curriculum Committee, rather than study the works of Marx, Weber and Durkheim, not to mention those of G. H. Mead in the United States and Norbert Elias in England and in the Netherlands, I insisted that we should study several plays: *The Tempest* (Shakespeare), *Our Town* (Thornton Wilder) and *Antigone* (Sophocles). I had in mind that we would focus on trauma and sibling relations, the matrix and equivalence, and gender and sexual identity, respectively. In my view these topics were at the heart of the group analytical project, and involved the integration of psychoanalysis and sociology. I also wanted us to explore personifications and interpretations as opposed to valences and role suction; the constraints and restraints of the foundation matrix and the dynamic matrix of social systems, or in other words the social unconscious; and the importance of the personality of each member of a group. Foulkes had yet to conceptualize the personal matrix, but this was "in the air" in London and in Lisbon.

The crucial issue was that we would and could change the world but not as we pleased! After all, the personal was political! Although roles could be interpreted by individual actors, the boundaries of roles could not be changed without challenging the dramatic structure of the play. An actor or a group who wished to mount such a challenge would be in difficulty with their audience, who would provide a kind of existential reflection of them.

Many senior colleagues thought that this was a luxury in a clinical training, especially for very busy psychiatrists and social workers who formed the core of our students or "candidates," the latter term conveying the political and religious origins of the role within the institution of psychotherapy itself. I argued that we could not afford not to include such a seminar in our training programs. I was greatly relieved that the students read the plays, and participated in our discussions of them in a way that was both lively and relevant to clinical work. I am the sole survivor of this seminar, but it was a foundational experience for us.

I am really delighted to have the opportunity of bringing back into our fold some of these ideas, interests and practices in the form of *Psychotherapeutic Playback Theater*. The subtitle of this book is *hall of mirrors on stage*. Although this notion of a hall of mirrors was adopted by Foulkes, Pines, Zinkin and others who were interested in mirroring in its normal and pathological forms, such work is not so much a hall of mirrors as it is a "chamber" of them, more of a room than a corridor, involving a myriad of looking glasses, some more reflective than others, some more opaque, some darker, some more truthful, some more securely fixed on the wall, etc. This is recognized by the authors of this seminal book. Therapeutic Playback Theater originated within the configuration of several interrelated disciplines, as did Group Analysis itself. It is hardly surprising that it should have begun to flourish in those societies and locations within them which are and have been most in flux, and in which people are most energetically and painfully searching for their collective and personal identities.

In the same way that social dreaming and dream telling has become an important part of Group Analysis, Psychotherapeutic Playback Theater is likely to become an important part of our practice and formation. It will be necessary to forge a format for this communication of lived experience in dramatic form, most probably something like the format used for "theatre in the round." Certainly, the boundaries between audiences and actors will be somewhat porous and negotiable! I would welcome such a development in our next conferences and workshops.

I am very appreciative of the contributions by the authors of this new book: Ronen Kowalsky, Nir Raz and Shoshi Keisari, with a chapter from Susana Pendzik. Originally published in Hebrew in 2019 by the Emily Sagol Arts Therapy Research Center at Haifa University, the manuscript was translated by Ami Atsmon and illustrated by Anna Ponomariova. Their book connects psychodrama, drama therapy and even art therapy with group analysis and other forms of psychoanalytical group therapy. It is an important contribution to the study and appreciation of the "in-between." I am happy to be able to include this work in the New International Library of Group Analysis. I enthusiastically commend it to both colleagues and students alike.

Earl Hopper
Series Editor

REFERENCES

Gorki, M. (2008). *The lower depths* (Tr. L. Irving). Middlesex: Wildhern Press.

Pirandello, L. (1995). *Six characters in search of an author and other plays* (Tr. and Intro. M. Musa). London: Penguin.

Roth, W.R. (2014). The birth of group analysis from the spirit of Theatre. *Group Analysis, 47*(3), 293–311.

Thompson, S. (1983). The group process in Chekhov's plays. In M. Pines (Ed.), *The evolution of group analysis* (pp. 344–358). London: Routledge and Kegan Paul. Reprinted London: Jessica Kingsley, 2000.

Wilke, G. (2021). What goes on between perpetrators, victims and bystanders in large groups. With Gerhard Wilke in conversation with Earl Hopper. IAGP Webinar – Zoom presentation, 17 April.

Learning TheraPlayback / Cheli Tal Shalem[1]

(Translation from Hebrew: Nisan Kowalsky)
Play–Back
To play,
To return the glory
After ending strikes a story –
Now, yesterday, in a midnight dream, tomorrow, years ago
(it's not my shame –
Others are to blame!)
And some unflattering pieces come together slowly, shadows
Sawn patch by patch, to a Peter Pan.
Forever young. Like me
Suddenly dancing
Like giant popping candy opens closes
See then the voices
To manifest, belittle, acclaim,
To willingly submit to un-control
Be the voice – Now! Now!
Who is the boss in here? Is it the road, or is it I who has to steer?
And it feels just the same
Until the story is also hers and also mine and also
A typo in the typography
(It's not an error
And even if it is
Mistakes are no big terror)
Then back to back they spin around
Burning on a spit and bound
And suddenly, the story has a different sound
So who is writing it? Who
Directs? Whose script is this?
Where does *will* then end, for desire to begin?
A Zoom-in transitions into zoom-Ouch!
And an understanding seeps in, perhaps a tear
Only, without the drama –
This all returns from age to age
And will return again
On stage

Note

1   Cheli Tal-Salem is an Israeli poet. "Learning TheraPlayback" is the title of the
    blog in which she documented her studies at the Institute of Psychotherapeutic
    Playback Theater.

Introduction – a house on the bridge

Ronen Kowalsky, Nir Raz, Shoshi Keisari

Psychotherapeutic Playback Theater can be envisioned as a bridge connecting two riverbanks: one is improvised theater that focuses on an individual's personal story; the other is the deep encounter between self and other within a psychoanalytically oriented group therapy process. Our recognition that this bridge is stable enough to build a house on and give life to a new therapeutic approach has been building gradually over the past 25 years, while we practiced Playback Theater, drama therapy, verbal psychotherapy (with individuals and groups), group analysis and theater. This is the first book to present Psychotherapeutic Playback Theater as a unique therapeutic field and discuss its theoretical foundations and the various considerations that inform conductors in choosing its diverse techniques and interventions.

Playback Theater is a theater genre in which a group of actors improvise a theatrical response to personal stories shared by audience members (Salas, 1993). Playback theater was first established in the 1970s in the United States, by *Jonathan Fox & Jo Salas*. They sought to establish a group that could create meaningful social theater that would bring together people and stories in a way that expanded the individual story through the other, by means of a theatrical improvisation that both mirrored and reinterpreted the story (Lubrani-Rolnik, 2009). In an interview, Fox defined Playback Theater as "a new type of theater that brings theater back from the field of entertainment to its earlier roots and purpose – preserving memory and holding the tribe together" (Fox, H., 2007, p. 92). Today, Playback Theater is commonly known and recognized as a prominent genre of improvisational theater in different communities throughout the world (IPTN, 2018).

Salas (1993) and Fox (1999) wanted to create a form of theater that would serve as a platform for promoting social change and hope, where the audience would not be mere passive spectators, but the heart of theatrical creation. They were inspired by the values of psychodrama, with which Fox was acquainted as a student of *Jacob Levy Moreno*, the founding father of psychodrama. However, while the founders of Playback Theater defined it as a theatrical approach that has curative potential (Salas, 2009), it was never explicitly presented or developed as a therapeutic method (Fox, 2007).

DOI: 10.4324/9781003167822-1

Although Playback Theater was originally defined as a non-therapeutic approach, many authors have pointed out the therapeutic potential of group processes in which the playback ritual plays a key role. Such processes offer an encounter with personal stories within a creative group process (Fox, 1999; Salas, 2007, 2009). For example, individuals coping with mental illness who participated in a Playback Theater course indicated, via self-report measures, higher levels of self-awareness, enjoyment and calm as well as increased ability to feel affinity and empathy toward other group members (Moran & Alon, 2011). Another study showed that a specialized Playback Theater group raised awareness of mental health issues, gave the audience an opportunity to share experiences of negative attitudes and discrimination regarding mental health labels and by that helped to decrease an experience of social distance (Yotis et al., 2017). A recent study validated the effect of a short-term group intervention, which integrates life review with Playback Theater participation, for improving various mental health indices among community-dwelling older adults including self-acceptance, personal growth, relationships with others, positive affect, meaning in life and self-esteem, as well as decreasing depressive symptoms. This improvement remained stable three months post-intervention (Keisari, Plagi et al., 2020). Another study explored a performative retelling group that was based on a variation of "restorative retelling" – an intervention focused on adaptation to traumatic bereavement – followed by a Playback Theater performance. This group helped to bridge the gap between law enforcement and formerly incarcerated citizens, improved attitudes toward ex-offenders and the police and increased meaning-making regarding life stressors (Smigelsky & Neimeyer, 2018).

By virtue of placing the personal story at the center of the group's creative process, Playback Theater became a popular tool among drama therapists, psychodrama therapists and group facilitators (Barak, 2013; Chesner, 2002; Keisari, Palgi et al., 2020; Keisari, Yaniv et al., 2018; Landy, 2006) and a regular part of the curriculum in leading creative arts therapies programs. These trends have led to the foundation of the Institute of Psychotherapeutic Playback Theater, which has been developing this new field of therapy since 2014. The institute publishes papers and materials, trains therapists and offers training programs for therapists from other approaches.

Psychotherapeutic Playback Theater takes place in the setting of a closed, ongoing group with a therapeutic contract, whose members share personal stories and "play back" each other's stories. Each member can be a teller, a player or an observer of the improvised theatrical response to the story (Kowalsky et al., 2019). In contrast with performance-oriented Playback Theater, which is a one-time show performed for an audience, in Psychotherapeutic Playback Theater, the group is seen as a social microcosm, which translates personal and group stories into the theatrical idiom. This idiom represents the manner in which different voices engage in dialogue in one's inner world (Kowalsky, 2014). In Psychotherapeutic Playback Theater, group members use dramatic play to resonate and expand the stories that arise in the group while the tellers witness these improvised responses. The personal experience introduced by the individual story becomes a collective experience, in which all group members take an active part.

The theatrical response utilizes diverse elements to offer new interpretations of the story, confronting the teller with its explicit and implicit aspects. The playing members resonate the materials of the story in the playing space[1] through images, archetypes, myths, universal stories, songs and other elements that the group's encounter with the story brings up. These resonances are presented as theatrical representations that expand the story, uncovering hidden meaning and making new discoveries (Pendzik, 2008). The theatrical response combines such theatrical representations to create a new, integrated piece that expresses the various aspects of the story and their potential (re)configurations.

Together with the interpretative space opened by group members around the story, the theatrical space of fantastic action represents a flexible approach to the use of dramatic tools in the therapeutic group space, drawing on the combination of improvisation and an encounter with personal material. The spatial positions of the different elements in the playing space, along with movement and music, create a theatrical aesthetic, which leads the spectator into the space of dramatic reality (Pendzik, 2006). This is a space where one can move between reality and imagination or between past, present and future and freely express and work through inner voices, feelings and thoughts. As a form of transitional space, dramatic reality enables unmediated observation of the teller's subjective experience.

Through our continuous work with Psychotherapeutic Playback Theater we have learned to appreciate its value as a teaching and practice method of psychoanalytic and group analytic concepts to psychotherapists in general. The embodiment of terms such as drive, object and object-relations, empathy and empathic failure, self-object, possible selves, positions, analytic third, container and contained, mirroring and exchange makes them tangible to a degree that one can "feel as if he is holding potential space in his hands," as one of our students put it. This tangibility gives therapists a unique chance to follow Bion's (1962) call for "Learning from Experience."

Psychotherapeutic Playback Theater has a special relationship with Group Analysis. It can be seen as a theatrical manifestation of *the tripartite matrix*, which Hopper (2020) has presented as the defining feature of Group Analysis and the way social systems ranging from states, societies, communities, organizations, families to actual groups are perceived and considered. The tripartite matrix also conceptualizes individuals as parts of social systems whose psyches are actually social systems (Hopper, 2003a, 2018).

The tripartite matrix consists of (1) *the personal matrix*, the relationships between the inner voices, which create the psyche of the individual (2) *the dynamic matrix*, the relationships between the members of a group or an organization and (3) *the foundation matrix*, the social and cultural contexts in which the group takes place. Hopper (2003a) emphasizes that these matrices are not separate entities but dynamic open systems, which maintain relations of reciprocity and simultaneity (Ahlin, 2019).

Every single element of the theatrical response contains simultaneously conscious and unconscious expressions of the three different matrices – the individual matrix of the story teller (as it is manifested in the presented narrative, and of the individual matrices of the playing members, as they are manifested in their interpretations), the dynamic matrix (as it is manifested through the theatrical expression of the relationships among the group members) and the foundation matrix (as it is manifested through the social and cultural layer, elements and context of the theatrical response).

It is possible to metaphorize the tripartite matrix as the system of relationships among cells of a body and between cells and the entire body. Each and every cell contains the genetic code of the entire body, but also serves a unique function in the body, therefore maintaining simultaneous relationships of similarity and uniqueness. Systemic fractals, borrowed from information and computer sciences, offer another metaphor. Systemic fractals represent the discovery that in many fields parts seem to manifest the same fundamental structure as their wholes (Hopper, 2003b).

We will demonstrate the way theatrical response is a materialization of the three matrices through a vignette documented by Keisari, Gesser-Edelsburg et al. (2020) in a Psychotherapeutic Playback Theater group with older adults, as part of research conducted in adult day centers in Israel. Simon, a 78-year-old man, shared with the group the loss of his younger brother. Simon's family immigrated to Israel from Egypt when he was 8 years old, and they were settled in a temporary immigrants' camp (Ma'abara). The Ma'abara is considered a traumatized chapter in Israeli history – In the early 50's massive immigration waves of holocaust survivors from Europe and Jews that fled from persecutions in Arab countries arrived in the young state. Housing and employment was scarce, and the enthusiastic immigrants were settled in temporary immigrant's camps, which became a synonym for poverty, unemployment and discrimination. This "temporary" housing solution, which actually resembled a refugee camp, continued into the early 60s. A few weeks after their arrival to Israel, Simon went out to play with his friends and failed to notice that his 2-year-old brother had left the tent and followed him. Later on, the brother was found dead in a pit. Simon described the guilt that accompanied him over the years, as a result of not being able to save his brother.

In response to his story, three female playing members volunteered to improvise three scenes from the story. The first scene focused on Simon's family after immigration with their hopes for a new life in Israel and traumatic disillusionment in the Ma'abara. The three playing members moved and danced on the playing space along a popular Israeli song, *Ach-Ya-Rab* (in

Arabic: Oh, dear god)[2] which was taken from a famous film *Sallah Shabati* –
an Israeli social satire, written by Ephraim Kishon about the chaos of Israeli immigration. The song written by Haim Hefer represents for many the
ambivalent experience of fulfilling the dream to immigrate to Israel and the
difficulties immigrates had in a country that is in the midst of absorbing
hundreds of thousands of Jewish refugees.

The second scene reflected the grief following the loss of Simon's brother.
The three playing members covered themselves with black fabrics. The teller
gave each one of them a role in the scene – his mother, his father and himself, and demonstrated the bereavement movements his mother use to do, as
beating their chests and heads. The playing members followed those movements, repeating sentences and sighing that reflected the guilt and grief of
Simon, his mother and father: "Ho God, how could this have happened that
I did not protect the baby! Bring my child back to me! Come back to me!"
The last scene focused on the growth of the family years later. The three
playing members held the fabrics in their arms as babies, looking at them
with love and admiration.

In the sharing circle, the three playing members shared with their own
stories from the Ma'abara, and the feeling of loss and guilt during the theatrical response. One of the women told about her immigration to Israel from
Argentina. She came as an individual in the 70s, a time of economical flour-
ishing in Israel, and not as a part of the immigration movement of the 50s.
She told the group that she feels as if she is lacking some knowledge of Israeli
life, but now she feels more a part of a common experience, as she feels a
connection with the other group members due to the stories they shared
with the group. Later, in the qualitative interview that was conducted with
the group members, Simon said:

> It was hard for me, but I had to tell this story because… it kept chasing
> me… and here (in the improvisation) no one said: "Why didn't you stop
> him from running away?" … no one (from the group) yelled at me …
> that set me free … because my whole life it has haunted me, the case.
> (I would ask myself): "Why did it have to happen and where did he go
> anyway?" Now, I think I realize that we couldn't have prevented it, there
> was nothing we could have done … I have no answer. It happened, and
> no one could stop it, and no one can bring him back to me.
> (Keisari, Gesser-Edelsburg et al., 2020, p. 11)

Considering the main images of the story and of the theatrical response –
the Ma'abara, the pit, the dead brother, the song, the blaming and grieving
women in black and the babies, one can see the way they are weaved from
the three matrices and that the therapeutic effect demonstrated in the vignette, and expressed in the comments of the teller and the group member,
is based on this tripartite fabric.

Looking through the personal matrix of Simon one can see the break-point of his life in his brother's meaningless death, expressed by the pit. This is connected in the song to the personal and foundation matrices character-ized by traumatic experience of losing the meaningfulness of immigration to Israel to the meaningless of day-to-day life of poverty and unemployment of the Ma'abara. The Ma'abara, the song and the pit simultaneously also em-body the feelings of alienation and wish to belong expressed by the playing member, reflecting her own personal matrix, the feelings of belonging and alienation among group members in the dynamic matrix and the trauma of alienation after the strong wishes to belong expressed in immigrating to Israel in the foundation matrix.

The images of the Ma'abara and the pit can also be seen as representing the old age day center as a sort of temporary immigrants' camp before death and the pit as representing fear of death. In a wider scope, the Ma'abara and the pit can be seen as representing in general situations of transformation and the anxiety related to being in a liminal state. The blaming and grieving women in black can be seen as embodying inner voices in Simon's personal matrix, fixating his mourning process, but also voices in the dynamic ma-trix of blaming oneself and one another in the feelings of alienation and mourning the loss of fantasy of oneness. In the foundation matrix this image has a strong resemblance to the lament women – representing the obliga-tion to mourn and the feelings of guilt over getting out of mourning. In this sense, the simultaneous decision of three female group members to play is very meaningful since Simon's guilt was embodied in the heavy mourning of his mother in the personal matrix and the lament women association in the foundation matrix. The image of the babies weaves all the images to-gether, and in this sense, all the three matrices together – bringing a wider perspective to the personal theme of guilt about a meaningless death, and to the group and social themes of the trauma of exclusion and fear of death. The image of the babies connects the lonely, bound to die, individual to the human intergenerational tapestry. This is done actually by tying the themes of the three matrices together, and thereby giving the individual a wider group and social meaning. Thus, the recognition of the tripartite matrix can be seen as having therapeutic value in itself.

The theatrical embodiment of images in Psychotherapeutic Playback Theater representing the tripartite matrix makes the connection among the three matrices tangible, enables working through of them in the playing space and widening of the group discussion and experience.

This book presents the fundamental principles of Psychotherapeutic Playback Theater with groups. It combines descriptions of this technique, alongside different variations and the conceptualization of the conductor's considerations in structuring the sessions and the group process. These descriptions are interlaced with reflections on the emerging psychothera-peutic process and discussions of the different psychoanalytic outlooks that inform its understanding. This newborn infant stands on the shoulders of giants, drawing on many sources of growth and inspiration. We believe that, by grounding this method in diverse theories, we are heeding the essential ethical call to develop through the other, which is at the very heart of Psychotherapeutic Playback Theater: development stems from recognizing the value of being part of a shared human tapestry.

The underlying thinking of Psychotherapeutic Playback Theater can be likened to a spool of thread – much like the reel of string Freud's grandson used for his Fort-Da game (Freud, 1920).[3] Every concept, every moment of interaction is multi-layered, inviting a variety of interrelated perspectives. In writing this book, we had to disentangle thread after thread and spread out, in a linear fashion, subjects that are not essentially differentiated or distinct. Naturally, we ended up with some loose threads. Because the understanding of certain subjects requires the reader to cover other subjects explained in different parts of the book, we added internal references directing the reader to those sections, to ensure a thorough understanding of each concept. We tried to keep these references to a minimum, so as not to disturb the flow of reading. At the same time, in an attempt to accommodate less methodic and chronological reading, each of the book's chapters entails at least minimal explanations of core concepts. Therefore, some parts may feel somewhat repetitive, as the same concepts are explained briefly in some places and more extensively and deeply in others.

Notes

1 We use the term "playing space" (two words) for the space in which the theatrical response takes place. Although it shares the same ethics with Johnson (2009) DVT's "playspace" (one word), it does have some different qualities, especially regarding the different possible relations with the spectators discussed in Chapter 6. Therefore, we preferred to use a slightly different term. We chose to use a verb and not a noun in order to emphasize the reoccurring creation of this space as an outcome of the playing activity within in a similar manner to Winnicott's (1971) potential space.

2 English translation extracted from http://hebrewsongs.com/?song=achyarab.

3 In "Beyond the Pleasure Principle" (1920), Freud describes his grandson playing with a wooden reel that has a piece of string tied to it. Holding onto the end of the string, the boy would throw the reel out of his bed and shout "*Fort!*" ("Gone!" in German) and then pull it back, shouting "*Da!*" ("There!"). Freud uses this example to discuss the therapeutic value of play-related activity as a metaphoric expression of anxiety-provoking material, which is worked through by the attempt to control it. In this case, according to Freud, the anxiety involved the disappearance and reappearance of his grandson's mother.

Chapter I

The story

A picture from the photo album of the mind

Ronen Kowalsky, Nir Raz, Shoshi Keisari

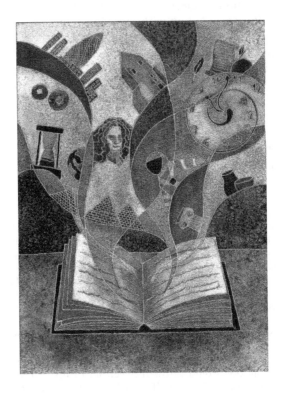

Figure 1.1

People tell stories. They use them to explain their lives to themselves and others. Self-identity develops as a story, which features places and times, a plot, characters and central themes. One's life story may be based on biographical facts, but it is interwoven with interpretations, cultural influences, associations and connections, culminating in the creation of a coherent

DOI: 10.4324/9781003167822-2

internalized myth of the self, whose very existence provides one's life with meaning. A coherent internalized life story allows the individual to live a life of purpose and supports the formation of a positive identity (McAdams, 2001). This chapter discusses the personal story and the way it is retold within the context of the shared experience of Psychotherapeutic Playback Theater.

Human experience is organized in the form of stories and the capacity for storytelling is thus the key to understanding the world (Bruner, 1990). The self emerges through the act of storytelling and our self-perception is shaped by the stories we tell ourselves and those that others tell about us (Schafer, 1983). Stories of the past – including one's personal story – create the meaning of one's life, both in the present and regarding one's expectations of the future. The interweaving of experiences and events captures a thematic pattern, which represents the individual's interpretation of the meaning of their life (Rosenthal, 1993).

People share important autobiographical memories with one another, carefully choosing to tell those stories which help them explain and present themselves. This process has a reciprocal influence on both the teller and the listener, as the telling of a memory naturally gives rise to insights and meaning in both parties (Bruner, 2004). This intersubjective encounter and the emerging dialogue create a space for the development of meaning and insight, influencing the emerging story and, through it, the manner in which both teller and listener construct their social identity (Gergen, 1991; Gergen & Gergen, 1988).

Thus, the story's essence is flexible, dynamic and adapted to the place and time in which it is being told. At the same time, it is also aimed toward the future (Barclay, 1994). Because the nature of a person's life story is dynamic, developing in accordance with their emerging identity and the different social situations they encounter (Gergen & Gergen, 1988; Greimas, 1991), it is only natural that, as it is repeatedly told and retold over time, this story is revised and reconstructed again and again. This dynamic quality also makes it possible to help an individual reconstruct their life story in a way that is better suited to and more effective for their developing self. Such a reconstructed story should expand one's perspective, enabling new discoveries for both teller and listener.

Yaniv, a 32-year-old man, tells the group that he is about to get married and, as his wedding day approaches, he finds himself increasingly withdrawn and consumed by profound sadness and confusion. He shares that he had felt a great deal of joy and wholeness in his relationship with his partner, until the moment they decided to get married – though both of them had felt that this decision was right and natural at the time. "It's as if there's something inside me that won't let me be happy, to partake in the experience of togetherness. I don't understand myself. It's supposed to be the most beautiful and meaningful moment of my life." Later on, to illustrate this, he tells the group about a weekend he spent with his partner at his parents and gets carried away in lengthy depictions of the pastoral farmland in which he grew up and the great atmosphere at his parents' place. He recalls driving a tractor through the fields of the small town as a teenager and how everything felt perfect back then. Yaniv talks about how tight-knit his family felt, about looking forward to celebrating birthdays and holidays together, about a special sense of esprit de corps surrounding his belonging to his family and the small town's community. He adds that he feels very open with his parents and tends to consult them about every major life decision he makes. He also adds that, when that weekend was over, he found it difficult to leave his parents' house.

By observing the story, the pastoral portrayal of Yaniv's childhood environment and his idyllic family atmosphere contextualizes the impending wedding. The latter symbolizes his final departure from his childhood home, the establishment of his own nuclear family and the need to confront his changing identity. From an identity that relies on being a "small town boy" and his parents' son, with all the esprit de corps these entail, he is now shifting to being an adult, with his own intrinsic identity and self-worth. In this sense, his decision to present this story to the Psychotherapeutic Playback Theater group can be seen as a kind of unconscious request that the group accompany him in his process of separating from his family of origin.

Each culture has its own stories, whose function is to preserve community identity and cohesiveness as well as to serve as means of entertainment, education and transmission of values. In all early human civilizations, stories helped to clarify human existence, convey knowledge, teach people about their tribal roles and facilitate the internalization of social norms. These stories were handed down from generation to generation in the tribe, through recollection and imitation. The earliest manifestations of storytelling included a variety of gestures and expressions. For example, pre-historic cultures painted on their cave walls symbols from the stories they heard, in an attempt to help the storyteller remember the story and pass it on. In later eras, the story was passed on by means of a narrative that included verbal, auditory (musical), visual (cave paintings) and movement (dance) aspects. Gestures, such as throwing sand in the air, using leaves and making wood carvings, were used to help the teller illustrate certain parts of the story, build tension and create drama. In this way, the verbal narrative became imbued with additional types of artistic expression, including theater; after all, as Shakespeare put it, "all the world's a stage, and all the men and women merely players…" (Shakespeare 1603/2009, set II).

In the 21st century, stories are still at the heart of human existence. In addition to the personal, social and cultural discourse expressed in literature, theater, film and journalism, personal stories are passed on via digital media, the internet and social networks (by posting on social media platforms, such as Facebook and Instagram, or sharing one's story on instant messaging apps). It is important to note that most social sciences approaches do not differentiate between the concepts of "narrative" and "story" (Riessman, 2008). This chapter focuses on personal narrative and the concept through which we chose to describe the processes related to its construction in Psychotherapeutic Playback Theater is the *personal story*.

Every story must have the elements of a dramatic scene: scenery, plot, protagonists, secondary characters, conflicts and resolutions. One's life story is constructed for an audience, whether external, such as friends and family members, or internal, like the super-ego, an internalized attachment object or God (McAdams, 2001; Polkinghorne, 1988). This basic assumption makes the introduction of one's story into theatrical and dramatic space a very natural and necessary process.

In Psychotherapeutic Playback Theater, the teller's personal story becomes a story in which all group members are involved and to which they all respond. The other members listen to the story with empathy and respond to it in a creative, improvised manner. They witness the telling and then resonate the mental and emotional materials to which it gives rise within them. In the playing space, the story takes on a life of its own: its different aspects become tangible and the teller becomes an observer of their own story, a witness to their own personal experience. This position grants them a new perspective, from which they can observe and explore the story, while maintaining aesthetic distance (Keisari, 2021; Keisari, Yaniv et al., 2018). The story expands through its encounter with others, as the playing members help the teller-observer discover new meanings and points of view.

This is illustrated through the theatrical response the group presented in response to Yaniv's story. The conductor asked Yaniv to choose a member who will play his role and that member then entered the playing space along with two others. Other member plays the song *Cheek to Cheek* by Louis Armstrong in the background, its opening line – "Heaven, I'm in heaven" – sounding throughout the playing space. The three playing members moved through the playing space huddled together, performing dance moves that involved a great deal of skin-to-skin contact. They smiled at each other, giving the impression that they have a good connection and that they are merged with each other. After about 30 seconds, a fourth member entered the playing space and stood at its other end. She and "Yaniv" made eye contact and smiled at each other. The two members who were dancing with Yaniv's character kept dancing as they did before, but his movement gradually changed. Every now and again, he stepped out to dance with the figure standing on the sideline and then came back to them. Little by little, his movement became less smooth and he seemed increasingly confused and torn between the two dances. At some point, he stopped, stood between these two "options" and reached out his arms to both sides, trying with all his might to grab hold of both at the same time – but to no avail. After the theatrical response was concluded, Yaniv said that he could see the different feelings he experienced in the situation he described. He added that images from his childhood room at his parents' house came to him and that he felt close to tears. During the sharing circle, the other members brought up stories from their own lives surrounding significant moments of development, in which they experienced "growing pains" and realized that development is not possible without a certain degree of separation and relinquishment.

The photo album of the mind

In this section, we examine what happens to the psychic material of the story when submitted to the creative group process of Psychotherapeutic Playback Theater. Human experience is, unsurprisingly, vaster than any story that seeks to capture it. Lived experience contains thoughts, feelings, tastes and smells, values, points of view and meanings which are never fully and exhaustively expressed in any given verbal story. The personal story can be seen as a picture in one's mental photo album. The teller leafs through their personal album and chooses a single picture. It may be an old black-and-white photograph which carries memories, smells, tastes and feelings. The teller offers us a tour, a glimpse into their inner world.

At this stage, our role as conductors is to help the teller focus on a certain part of the photo they chose. This process allows careful observation of each and every detail: the background, the landscape, the characters and their relationships, objects, facial expressions, body positions, atmosphere, emotions, etc. The aim of this process is to bring the picture to life by exposing new colors and details, emphasizing pre-existing elements, expanding its present limits and discovering new elements. Finally, all the details need to be combined in order to create a new, integrated picture, which holds both the pre-existing and the newly discovered elements. This new picture is re-inserted into the personal photo album, more integrated through the insights gained in the Psychotherapeutic Playback Theater process and freshly colored with the qualities of acceptance, sharing, listening and presence. It is as if the teller has come back from a long journey, during which he collected various souvenirs, experiences and gifts – new shades, additional perspectives and the qualities of a deep, interpersonal encounter. Taken together, these newfound elements have imbued the teller's pre-existing experience with a new light.

In Yaniv's story, one can see how the theatrical response presents his relationships with his parents and his partner from a novel perspective, which highlights the pain he is feeling in the process of separating from his parents as the key difficulty surrounding his upcoming marriage. This clarification is an initial step toward the change that needs to happen in Yaniv's view of his relationship with his parents in order to facilitate his further development as an individual and the formation of his own nuclear family.

The journey of the personal story

The main focus of this chapter is the exploration of the different stages in the journey of the personal story – starting with its transition from the teller to the playing space and, through the Psychotherapeutic Playback Theater group process, back to the teller: (1) *selection* – the story that is chosen to come to light emerges as a result of particular motives and needs; (2) *the theatrical response* – responds to the story and contains several components: theatrical mirroring of the story's conscious parts, the deconstruction of the narrative into different elements and, finally, their reintegration into a new, complete structure; (3) *back to the teller* – after the theatrical response, the teller responds by sharing any thoughts and feelings that arose during the response; (4) *the sharing circle* – group members share personal stories which came up in response to the story or the feelings they experienced during the theatrical response and (5) *the red thread* – the conductor recapitulates the various stories and responses and proposes an interpretation designed to tie them all together.

Choosing the story that asks to "come to light"

In Psychotherapeutic Playback Theater groups, members are invited to share their personal stories. The stories presented to the group are the starting point of the therapeutic process, providing the necessary materials for dramatic response. As the group process unfolds, stories begin to touch on deeper and deeper issues and the group's creative processing becomes more meaningful for both the teller and the other members. Members use their stories to present their inner world, their motives, the ways in which they define their identity and the choices that give their lives direction and meaning. These stories create a sense of continuity and tie together past, present and future. They often contain internal conflicts, feelings of lack or longing, inhibitions or obstacles to one's desire to act and conflicting emotions.

A study conducted on a sample of 27 elderly members in a Psychotherapeutic Playback Theater group found that 16 members shared stories that focused on unresolved issues from their past (Keisari, Gesser-Edelsburg et al., 2020). Group members oscillated between wanting to share themselves and their experiences with the group and explore their stories as a path for growth and development and having difficulties sharing feelings of pain, vulnerability and weakness and worrying that such exposure will have a negative outcome. As the group progressed, members felt safer, dared to share increasingly personal stories with the group and were better able to rely on the safety of the group space in coping with difficult life events, pain, vulnerability and weakness. In this manner, they were able to achieve personal growth and development.

The playing space, where the personal story is revealed before the group, creates a shared experience that enables the teller to face difficult feelings of loneliness and alienation and embrace feelings of solidarity, containment and empathic presence. Group members become fully involved in the teller's story and their identification with it facilitates the normalization of the teller's experience. As their experience is being acknowledged by those around them, the teller feels a sense of solidarity. This feeling is accompanied by a sense of universality, resulting from the teller's recognition that the experiences, feelings, emotions and difficulties they expressed are common to everyone. Yalom and Leszcz (1995) define this experience of universality as one of the curative factors in group therapy, allowing members to feel connected to the world and have a sense of belonging to the greater family of humanity. This often results in feelings of relief and an increase in one's ability to receive help from others. When a story that contains vulnerability and conflict comes to light, the teller is allowing the other group members to help them carry the heavy burden which they have so far carried alone. One member described this experience as follows: "in the group, we often share stories that have made us feel outside the realm of what is human [...] Playback brings us back into the fold, making us human again."

It is important to note that the movement between the desire and the need to share and the fear of exposure and vulnerability is a regular part of the process. Both the group and the individual member (the teller) oscillate between paralyzing anxiety and the desire for intimacy (Biran, 2015a). At this stage, the teller's greatest concern is whether the other members will be able to bear the weight of their story along with them. This concern is often accompanied by feelings of guilt and questions such as "maybe the burden I've asked the group to shoulder is too heavy?" Other inner voices emerge: "I knew I shouldn't have told them." Later in this chapter, we will discuss the possibilities embodied in the Psychotherapeutic Playback Theater process and the means by which the story – often experienced by the teller as a "millstone around their neck" – may be perceived in a new, sometimes transformative light.

When the story is processed through the theatrical response, the other members encounter it, respond to it and share similar experiences. In this way, a new, shared experience is created; a new layer envelops the existing story, assimilates the old memory and becomes a part of it. This new experience promotes transformation and enables personal growth for the teller and the other group members (Keisari et al., 2018; Keisari, Gesser-Edelsburg et al., 2020; Keisari, Palgi et al., 2020). For example, Yaniv's story was shared at a rather advanced stage of the group process. Because it was not a "presentable" story but one told in a confused manner and evoking implicit material, his story even served as a kind of turning point. This transition is manifest in the correspondence between the contents of the personal story, which concern the unsettling of identity, and the group process, in which stories involving experiences of awkwardness and even shame are being introduced into the playing space.

The theatrical response

The theater improvisation presented in response to the story comprises three main components: *mirroring, deconstruction* and *reconstruction*. All three aspects are always present in the theatrical response, though their relative proportions may change, depending on the story, the teller and the group process.

Theatrical mirroring

This component entails the group's engagement with the overt and conscious parts of the story. Theatrical mirroring is based on the psychoanalytic concept of *mirroring*. In this part of the response process, playing members focus on expressing and validating the teller's conscious experience. It is important for the teller to be able to identify with their story on the level of content and narrative. The goal of the playing members is to present the teller's conscious experience by mirroring the various milestones of their unfolding narrative. Even more important is emotional mirroring, by which the playing members express, elucidate and acknowledge the emotions the teller experienced throughout the story. Most importantly, the mirroring part of the response must not reject the teller's experience but provide additional points of view. Through it, the teller recognizes and acknowledges his story and his emotional experience is validated. In the above example, this is evident in the manner in which the theatrical response mirrored Yaniv's story on both the narrative and emotional levels. On the former, the playing members chose a form that mirrored the different characters in his story and his respective relationships with them. On the latter, the theatrical response mirrored the feelings of confusion clearly present in his story, so that Yaniv would be able to recognize himself and have his feelings validated. Finally, the mirroring component of the theatrical response is essential in Psychotherapeutic Playback Theater, as it paves the way for other, more interpretative components and allows the teller to broaden the range of experiences they accept as relevant. The therapeutic significance and additional aspects of the theatrical mirroring will be discussed in further detail in the next chapter.

Deconstruction

After mirroring the teller's overt, conscious experience, it is time to express their inner voices, feelings and emotions. The group now takes the different parts of the picture and divides them into discrete elements representing the different voices in the story. This idea is inspired by White and Epston's (1990) principles of *narrative therapy*. According to this approach, the life of the patient is controlled by a dominant story which exerts it power by dictating how the issues related to the person's identity and choices are framed. In such cases, the dominant story often maintains its hold over the teller's identity by limiting their openness to perceiving other points of view. When the dominant story has such a negative influence, the construction of a new story is advised (White, 2007). The concept of "re-authoring" the story drives the therapeutic process (Murray et al., 1992; Ricks et al., 2014) in a way that enables the deconstruction and reconstruction of its components.

Yaniv consciously chose to share with the group his story about feeling sad and confused about his upcoming marriage. His descriptions of his broader familial context are presented not as part of the story he intended to tell, but as associations, a kind of general air and background for his pre-nuptial confusion. The theatrical response re-edits the story by deconstructing it into two main components: Yaniv's relationship with his family of origins and his feelings toward his partner. It makes room for the theatrical exploration of each of these components in turn. Later on, this will fuel the process of reconstruction, which will reposition these distinct components on a single stage and explore their relationship.

The narrative therapy approach expresses narrative thinking in several ways. First, present life experiences are connected to past memories in a way that facilitates the emergence of new meaning. Second, re-describing events in a linear manner creates beginning and end points, which help establish a coherent inner experience and thus a more unified and coherent sense of self. Finally, the presentation of multiple perspectives and interpretations expands the range of possible perceptions of one's life story and its potential meanings (Keisari, 2021). This, in turn, enables the development of a flexible, creative and spontaneous outlook on lived situations in real time (White and Epston, 1990). In many ways, the instrument of the theatrical response can be seen to apply these aspects of narrative therapy: it maintains the individual's position as the active protagonist of their own story; it lays out the story's different components and presents their concrete theatrical enactment as an integrated whole, which captures and restructures the story as the sum of its parts; and it does all this with the help and support of others.

In addition to offering a tangible experience and exploring different perspectives of the narrative, the deconstruction of the story allows the clear expression of voices of different parts of the self: ego, super-ego and id; drive and obstacle; object-relations; fantasy and reality. Each psychic element can be represented by a separate theatrical element: the emotional qualities, the emerging imagery and the forms and perspectives of the various characters. Deconstructing the story allows us to highlight the expression of inner voices or other figures in the story. For example, if the story is about a mother-son relationship and playing members notice the guilt experienced by either the son or the mother, they can present the voice of guilt. Moreover, the different elements of the theatrical response express the internal experience of both the teller and the playing members. Such externalizing expression alleviates the sense that one's experience is withdrawn, suppressed and onerous.

In Psychotherapeutic Playback Theater, the theatrical response uses the language of imagery and symbols, which is akin to the language of dreams. This language allows the application of two important skills: *distancing* and *expansion*.

The element of distancing is already present in the most primary setting of Psychotherapeutic Playback Theater, in which the teller observes his personal experience from the sidelines, without participating in it or directing it (J. Fox, 2007). During the theatrical response, the playing members make a point of not looking at the teller, in order to allow them to engage in distanced observation of presented material. Psychotherapeutic Playback Theater also uses distancing to explore past experience in the "here and now." Further distancing may be achieved by transporting the personal story to some parallel place or time, by bringing to the playing space corresponding images and associations from the world of fairytales, biblical stories, myths, etc. In this way, the story achieves "amplification" (Jung, 1947/1960), meaning that it is connected to a continuum of cultural and historical wisdom. This connection expands it beyond its concrete limitations, imbues it with new meaning and gives the teller a renewed sense of belonging to the human race and its history. Within narrative space, we move between *proximity* to the story – to the personal experience expressed by the teller and empathically reconstructed by the playing members – to *distance* from the story, which leads to fantastic times, places and spaces. Distancing enables the teller to observe psychic material that involves a great deal of vulnerability and pain from a more emotionally safe position.

In the theatrical response responding to Yaniv's story, the use of abstract, movement-based expression moved beyond the realm of the concrete story and created the experience of distancing that allowed the teller to observe his story from a new vantage point. Distancing allowed Yaniv and the other members to depart from the concrete exploration of the upcoming marriage and address the broader theme of developmental transitions and the struggles they entail.

In Psychotherapeutic Playback Theater, distancing also coincides with the therapeutic factor of "externalizing the problem," as defined by White and Epston (1990). One of the main elements in narrative therapy, the principle of "externalizing the problem" allows the individual to recognize their abilities to cope with challenging aspects and issues defined as problems. By positioning the "problem" as external to them, the individual separates it from their identity, regaining a sense of power and control. Theatrical response in Psychotherapeutic Playback Theater can reposition the problem as external to the teller, using dramatic representation to render it more distant but just as tangible. The teller can then observe the problem, explore it and gain deeper knowledge of it from a safer, more empathic standpoint, while supported by the conductor and the group.

In addition, the theatrical response enables the concrete expression of the individual's strengths. This reconceptualizes the situation as belonging to the realm of "unique outcomes" (White and Epston, 1990). These different aspects of distancing, as embodied in the theatrical response in Psychotherapeutic Playback Theater, reinforce the coping potential of both the teller and the group members.

Expansion means working in *surplus reality* (Moreno, 1963) or *dramatic reality* (Pendzik, 2006) to create a flexible space in which performers can jump from place to place, time to time, fantasy to reality. It means providing a new perspective on the story, by expanding its reality and drawing on its hidden unconscious dimensions, which are seldom fully experienced or expressed in everyday life. In the *surplus* or *dramatic* reality of the playing space, playing members can express inner voices and thoughts, shift back and forth in time by playing a scene from the past or the future, meet people the teller never met or people who are no longer part of their life. Such surplus maneuvers allow the teller to actually experience the events anew, while engaged in a process of reflection and gaining insight (Moreno & Moreno, 1969).

The theatrical response includes various elements capable of generating new interpretations and confronting the teller with various explicit and implicit facets of their story. In addition to surplus maneuvers, playing members resonate the story's materials in the playing space by introducing images, archetypes, myths, universal stories, poems and other elements that arise in the encounter between the group and the story. These resonances also serve to expand the story, revealing new meanings and unexpected elements (Pendzik, 2008).

In the theatrical response to Yaniv's story, the use of the popular song *Cheek to Cheek* created a kind of imaginary heavenly backdrop, against which the story was presented in an abstract, movement-based idiom. This allowed the group to link the personal story with the archetypal and universal theme of "leaving paradise," thus facilitating a broader outlook on the story's theme as well as creating an associative and emotional connection between the teller and the other group members.

Reconstruction

The theatrical response in Psychotherapeutic Playback Theater combines different elements to create a new, integrated picture which presents the various aspects of the story and the different ways these can come together. The theatrical response can utilize different dramatic structures, which represent a single, isolated component through certain theatrical images (sound and movement), intensify it and position it within the playing space, culminating in an integrative combination of all elements together. This process generates a new picture, reconstructing the story. The theatrical response created by the group in response to Yaniv's story deconstructed and reconstructed his story. It presented the relations between the different parts of the story by positioning them on a single stage, which became a representation of Yaniv's inner world. This elucidated the unconscious conflict Yaniv had sensed and highlighted the role of his familial context in his emotional state. The group thus shifted the focus from his feelings of confusion and sadness about the upcoming marriage to his difficulties with separating from his family of origins. The group discussion that followed the theatrical response revolved around difficulty with separation and the need to resolve it in order to allow for growth. In fact, this discussion presented Yaniv's confusion about his marriage as a symptom of a broader difficulty concerning his process of separating from his family and his need to complete this process to be able to build a family of his own.

The deconstruction and reconstruction of the story take place within an aesthetic framework, which uses the playing space in accordance with the story's emotional content. For example, more conscious psychic materials are presented *downstage*, while less conscious materials are presented *upstage*. Theatrical aesthetics facilitate a formal kind of observation, which simultaneously resonates the internal structure of different parts of the mind and their restructuring. In establishing the aesthetic framework, one can use creative elements from the realms of theater, movement and music and utilize objects and pieces of cloth, which are imbued with the psychic materials of the story.

During the theatrical response, different aspects of the story are presented. Those taking part in this process – the teller, the playing members and the observing members – intuitively link these different aspects by attending the variety of voices presented and organized within the playing space. Members thus engage in processes of analysis and synthesis: *analysis* involves the deconstruction of the story into its constituent elements; *synthesis* is the process of integrating these constituent elements through different kinds of theatrical expression.

This highlights the great importance of presenting each and every voice and aspect of the story in the playing space in a discrete, isolated way. In this way, the theatrical response validates the teller's experience. For example, when showing a conflict, each side should be presented in a clear and distinct manner. Voices that simultaneously express both sides of the conflict are likely to increase confusion and obscure the expression of the conflict in the theatrical response. On the other hand, the creation of clear, externalized voices, which present opposing and unmitigated views, elucidates the conflict and helps the teller make sense of it. This is possible because the playing space is holding the different voices together for the teller, allowing them to recognize the influence this conflict has over them. This type of picture expresses itself as a whole that is greater than the sum of its parts.

Bringing the story back to the teller

Once the theatrical response is over, the playing members remain in the playing space and turn to look at the teller. This is a symbolic act which brings the story back to him. At this stage of the process, the memory from their photo album is returned to the teller, having been imbued with new interpretations and new discoveries of hitherto unknown shades of color and meaning. The conductor then turns to the teller and gives them a chance to respond to the group's performance. The conductor encourages the teller to share whatever thoughts and feelings came up while watching the theatrical response. The teller may comment on the parts of the theatrical response that they experienced as validating their initial experience or note the parts they felt moved too far away from this experience. This type of sharing is an important part of the therapeutic process. It allows the teller to express, specify and name their experience as well as what they need – from the group or from themselves – providing an opening for further growth and development.

After attending the teller's feedback, the conductor may suggest that the group create another theatrical response. Any material that came up in the discussion and any needs indicated by teller's observations are integrated and mirrored in this "follow-up" response. The function of this part of the process is to "give the story back" to the teller – along with a feeling of greater control over their story, in a manner that reinforces a sense of separation and autonomy in their relationship with the group. This therapeutic intervention is especially significant in cases where the experience conveyed by the story suggests feelings of lack of control, helplessness, over-dependence or difficulty with separation.

The sharing circle

The next stage in the process is the sharing circle, in which group members verbally share personal stories which came up throughout their encounter with the teller's story and the theatrical response. The discussion that takes place in the sharing circle allows playing members to process the experience they have just embodied and resonate emotional contents from the story. The sharing circle, therefore, enables them to "de-role," to leave their designated theatrical roles and observe the process from a personal and more separate perspective. The sharing circle is an inherent and important part of the therapeutic process. It creates a shared experience in which all group members – the teller, the playing members, the witnessing members and the conductor – have a place and a role. Processing the experience, observing it and being able to make room for the additional material it gives rise to are all essential components of the global experience of the Psychotherapeutic Playback Theater process.

The sharing circle creates a space in which members can once again find their own individual voice, recognize the similarities and differences between themselves and others and understand and support each other, both despite and because of such differences (Yalom & Leszcz, 1995). In the context of psychodrama, Moreno et al. (2013) claimed that the sharing circle embodies the main therapeutic effect of the psychodramatic process – the emergence of empathy among group members and its enhancement by means of the individual protagonist/teller. Accordingly, the different psychodramatic components – doubling, the alter ego, sociometry and even the catharsis of the protagonist within and in front of the group – are all aimed at achieving this goal.

At this stage, members can introduce any of their own personal stories that came up during the process. Playing members can share feelings and thoughts about the creative process itself and what they discovered through it – about the role they played, the choice whether to play or to observe, transformations that occurred through play and interactions with other members in the playing space. At this point, one may and should perceive the creative process as a way of observing transference processes. Thus, when a member shares his experience of being dumbstruck in the playing space, feeling detached and blank during the theatrical response, this may be indicative of the teller's experience, may hint at hidden layers of the story and attest to the encounter between the playing member's inner world and the themes of the story. It is important to encourage playing members not to ignore inner voices that arise during the creative process and, instead, to consider them as significant to the transference process emerging around, toward and within the story. For example, when a playing member feels stuck and keeps drawing a blank during the response or if they feel anxious or ashamed about the creative process, it is important that they express these feelings and note how they relate to their encounter with the story's contents.

At this stage, it is important to keep the focus on observation. Group members often feel the need to offer the teller advice, encouragement and support. However, this reassuring attitude may keep them from accessing and expressing the personal experiences that came up in their encounter with the story. Therefore, the conductor's role at this point is to guide members to relate to the story on a personal level and avoid giving advice or recommending solutions. The sharing of personal experiences normalizes the teller's experience, maintains the shared experience and transforms it from an individual experience into a universally human experience. This aspect is of great therapeutic importance.

The sharing circle creates a balance within the group by changing its focus of exposure, from the teller to all group members. The *shared experience* is maintained, generating a deep sense of intimacy and giving rise to insights and understanding for all members. Processes of validation, normalization, recognition and appreciation of the teller's experience are still in effect and are now occurring on the group level.

Before it is shared, psychic material is felt as a heavy burden, both disproportionate and decontextualized. The process of re-listening to the story, during the theatrical response and the sharing circle, enables the group to share the weight of the teller's experience. This allows the teller to take in new dimensions, perspectives and contexts which, in turn, lead to personal development, growth and change. The group's ability to hold the story, to use it as raw material for its creative process and explore it together creates a container for the mental contents it entails. This process – which includes normalization and the transformation of personal material into something that is shared, known and containable by others – reduces the anxiety surrounding one's exposure, the encounter with the story's contents and related feelings of guilt and shame.

The red thread

In every Psychotherapeutic Playback Theater session, members choose to share personal stories, revealing pictures from the photo album of their mind. At a certain point, a common thread emerges, connecting all these stories and pictures and creating a page in the group's collective photo album. Every session is a new page in this album, comprising all the photos and themes raised by the group that day.

The stories emerging in any given session are often linked through some conceptual and/or emotional thread, which traces their shared elements and motifs. One story sparks another, as stories often arise in response to the themes of previous stories. This process, on the whole unconscious and unseen, has to do with feelings, thoughts and the way in which each story resonates with the other members who, as the session progresses, become tellers themselves. The red thread, which thematically and emotionally ties together the different stories, is a key aspect of the conductor's work. Discovering and defining this thread helps the conductor understand the central themes with which the group is preoccupied.

Group exercises for working with stories

Entering the role of the other

The group is divided into pairs. Each pair is divided into teller and listener. The teller then presents his or her story to the other group members. After they finish telling, the conductor invites the listener to present their partner's story in the first person. During their retelling, the conductor can interrupt them to ask questions. Once they are done, the conductor turns to the original teller and asks them to share their experience of witnessing this own story retold by someone else.

Deconstructing the story (five-sentence synopsis)

Members are asked to move around the room and think of a story that is on their mind. Then, they are asked to think about the story's specific sensory elements: smells, tastes, visual images, colors and feelings. The use of sense-memory allows members to delve deep into the emotional world of the images and characters inhabiting their story. Next, members are asked to write down their story in an automatic flow, without any self-censoring or attempts at structure. After they finish writing, they are asked to underline five sentences that represent the essence of their story's narrative, each sentence capturing one of the following, in order: beginning; underlying impulse/desire; obstacle; the plot's highlight or turning point; ending/resolution.

When listening to a story, members often feel a strong sense of responsibility and commitment not to miss a single detail. This attempt at total recall tends to make the response clumsy, overloaded and overwhelming. When presented with all the details of the story, it may seem impossible to choose and focus on the material one wants to present on stage. This exercise is designed to allow members to experience finding the crux of the story by choosing five sentences that constitute the story's core, essence and meaning. This exercise can be continued with the following technique.

Exposing the heart of the story through the "fluid sculpture" pattern

Members are divided into groups of four. One of them reads their five sentences to the other three, who then use the "fluid sculpture" pattern to create a theatrical response based on these sentences. One of the playing members expresses a movement that represents an element or a feeling that arises from one of the five sentences. After assuming a position, they freeze and form a sculpture and then recite the sentence they chose. The second playing member assumes a different position, freezes and recites a different sentence. The third one does the same. Finally, all three "frozen sculptures" are standing side by side and each playing member repeats their own sentence. At the end of the theatrical response, the teller shares whatever feelings and thoughts came up while watching and explains how the minimalism of the response influenced their experience.

This exercise illustrates the importance of aesthetic form, which acts as a container for the story's contents, as well as of focusing and paring down in order to reveal "the heart of the story." Finally, by sharing their experience of watching the theatrical response, the teller is promoting the emergence of new perspectives on the story.

Conclusion

The personal story is the heart of the Psychotherapeutic Playback Theater process. This chapter described the main components of the therapeutic process by which a personal story is brought "to light" in the group, given new interpretations through its encounter with others, enriched with new insights and perspectives and, through its reconstruction, transformed into a shared group experience. These components, which create an opportunity for both the teller and the other members to experience conceptual-emotional change, constitute significant therapeutic factors. Psychotherapeutic Playback Theater also involves other therapeutic factors, which are discussed in the following chapters. One key factor is theatrical mirroring, which is a meaningful component of the theatrical piece created in response to the personal story.

Chapter 2

Theatrical mirroring

Ronen Kowalsky, Nir Raz, Shoshi Keisari

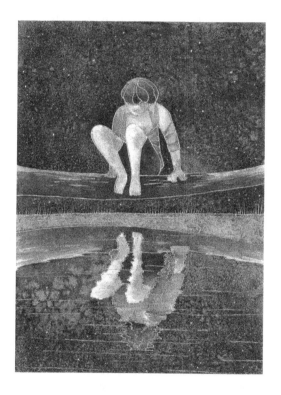

Figure 2.1

The focus of this chapter is theatrical mirroring, which is the most fundamental and significant component of the theatrical response in Psychotherapeutic Playback Theater. Theatrical mirroring can be seen as a way of mirroring the story back to the teller, as played by the group members. Grounded in the psychoanalytic notion of mirroring, theatrical

DOI: 10.4324/9781003167822-3

mirroring expands this notion by using dramatic language – characters, images, music and movement. Theatrical mirroring is a dramatic presentation of the more conscious parts of the story – its *overt* narrative and emotional aspects. We will examine how the theatrical response mirrors the story back to the teller, expressing parts of their story in ways that allow them to recognize themselves in it. Other aspects of the theatrical response, those which expand the response to the story beyond the explicit level and entail additional therapeutic interventions, will be presented in subsequent chapters.

Theatrical mirroring is the foundation of the group members' theatrical response, the core response to the personal story. As mentioned, it includes a significant and essential component of human relations – *mirroring*. The value of mirroring has been recognized in human civilization since antiquity and its important qualities are expressed in many myths and legends. The word "mirror" encompasses two simultaneous qualities: observation and wonder. The source of the word mirror is the French *miroir*, taken from the Latin root *mirare*, meaning "observation"; it is related to the verb *mirari*, which means "to wonder." These two qualities of the mirror are expressed in legends, fairytales, myths, dreams and the magical period of childhood (Pines, 1984). Pines (1985) also claims that the term "mirroring" contains an abundance of images: marvel, mirages, miracles; in other words, it expresses magical and wondrous capabilities. Consider the myth of Narcissus, who fell in love with his own reflection, or the mirror in Snow White, which reflects the truth the queen cannot bear and becomes the source of her aggression (Todar & Weinberg, 2006).

Moreover, mirroring is discussed extensively as an essential component of human development in psychoanalytic literature (Kohut, 1971; Lacan, 2001; Mahler, 1967; Winnicott, 1971) and many theoreticians have singled it out as possessing essential therapeutic qualities. Kohut (1971) found this element of particular importance to babies, who discover their reflection in their mother's eyes and are thus able to see themselves in all their splendor and glory. This cultivates a healthy narcissism, which is crucial for psychological development. At this stage (6–18 months), the infant – whose experience involves fragmentation and a lack of coordination, which are felt by the self as a lack of wholeness – is fascinated by this external, complete self-image, seen in the mirror of their mother's eyes. By perceiving this reflection, the infant begins to develop a notion of the self and a sense of coherence. Winnicott (1971) emphasizes how important it is for the mother's gaze to truly reflect the infant:

> The mother gazes at the baby in her arms, and the baby gazes at his mother's face and finds himself therein [...] provided that the mother is really looking at the unique, small, helpless being and not projecting her own expectations, fears, and plans for the child. In this case, the child

would find not himself in his mother's face, but rather the mother's own projections, the child would remain without a mirror and for the rest of his life would be seeking this mirror in vain.

(p. 112)

A "good-enough" mother reflects to her child feelings of love and omnipotence that are vital to its growth and development. Stern (1983) perceives mirroring as a formative experience for the self during its early stages of development, an experience through which mother and child create shared experiences (such as a mutual gaze, looking at something together, a mutual smile), where one reflects and echoes the other. According to Stern, this amazing discovery that the baby is making – that their experience is part of a whole spectrum of shared human experiences – serves as the foundation for establishing subjective intimacy and acknowledging separateness.

Another contribution reinforcing the importance of mirroring to human development was made in the 1990s, through the discovery of *mirror neurons*. The presence of these neurons can be seen in the fact that certain areas of the brain are activated both when an individual performs an action themselves and when they observe that actions being performed by others (Stueber, 2008). While the role of mirror neurons in our understanding of others is still unclear, this discovery suggests that human experience does not only draw on personal engagement, but it also draws on observing the experiences of others, as reflected in the brain's neural activity.

In addition to developmental theory and neuroscience, a key concept in the field of group therapy is Foulkes' (1964) notion of the *Hall of Mirrors*, which highlights the role of the mirroring processes taking place in the group in facilitating the members' development. The individual both sees himself mirrored in his interactions with the other group members and sees them respond the same way he does or in ways that differ from his behavior. In this manner – through his reflection in the eyes of the others – he comes to know himself. In this context, one should note that there are different types of mirrors: mirrors that enable modeling and imitation; empathic mirrors; validating mirrors; mirrors which offer growth-promoting confrontation; inverted mirrors and more (Schlapobersky, 2016). These different types of mirrors provide support, empathy and containment, while also instilling motivation for change, growth and development.

In a Psychotherapeutic Playback Theater group, Yaron, a 42-year-old man, shares a feeling of distress that arises in relation to his wife. He says that, several years before, she had made a significant professional transition, leaving a steady, high-income job, in which she felt boredom, emptiness and meaninglessness for a job she experiences as very meaningful and self-realizing. Yaron describes his decision to stand by her and support her during this transition. However, in the past year, her new line of work has been facing a serious crisis and her income has decreased substantially. She felt a sense of failure and Yaron describes her getting seriously depressed in a way that affected many aspects of their shared life, both as a couple and as parents. His wife's condition worsened after she had been offered a financially lucrative position in her old line of work. She has been obsessively deliberating between the two options, only capable of seeing their respective downsides. Yaron felt a great deal of helplessness and shared that all the things he had tried to do to alleviate her distress have been in vain.

> I tell her that she should stay in her present field and then she gets upset because she feels stuck there. I tell her to go back to her old profession and then she gets upset because she says that she felt suffocated there. I tell her that the only thing that matters to me is her happiness and then she gets upset because, at the moment, she's incapable of feeling happy and I'm only making her feel guilty about it.

In the theatrical response, the group chose to present different voices within an open improvisation. The first to enter the playing space was a group member who moved aimlessly in circles and expressed the teller's confusion and helplessness: "I don't know what I'm going to do, everything I do is wrong." Then, two other members entered the playing space – a man and a woman. The man got on his knees and told the woman repeatedly, "all I want is for you to be happy," while the woman replied, "But I'm not. You don't understand me." Then, the man repeated the words "I'm trying, I'm constantly trying," while slowly fading to silence; and the woman added: "do you love me when I'm not?" and then said, in masculine form, addressing a woman, "and you, do you love me when I'm not?" Another member paced back and forth in the back of the playing space, repeatedly saying to himself: "what does it say about me that I can't solve my wife's problem? What kind of husband am I? What kind of man am I?" The last playing member entered the playing space. She joined the playing member who was pacing back and forth upstage and said: "I need you to trust me. I don't trust myself and I need you to trust me."

This open improvisation shows how the group is providing Yaron with different kinds of mirrors, each one playing a different role. The performance of the first playing member, who expressed Yaron's helplessness and confusion, can be seen as an *empathic mirror* that validates his experience. The playing member who paced back and forth also offered an empathic mirror, but this one also broadened the perspective by pointing out the implications concerning Yaron's self-image as a husband and as a man. The response also entailed several *confronting mirrors*: the man pleading with his wife to be happy and the woman asking "do you love me when I'm not?" These mirrors reflect the sense of abandonment one can feel in response to a sentence that is seemingly supportive, such as "all I want is for you to be happy." Another confronting mirror can be seen in the loneliness exhibited by each of the characters in the playing space during this part of the response. Then, the entrance of the playing member who said, "I need you to trust me. I don't trust myself and I need you to trust me" and joined the pacing man presented Yaron with an *expanding mirror*, which may help him hold the confronting mirrors offered to him by encompassing the potential and the strengths of his relationship with his wife.

It is important to note that not all mirrors are positive. Theoretical literature describes negative mirrors as well. As mentioned, Winnicott (1971/1995) discusses malignant mirroring: if a mother is preoccupied with herself, for whatever reason, her mood will be reflected to the infant, teaching it to separate from the mother prematurely and to recognize the needs of the other before realizing and fulfilling her own. Eventually, this relinquishment of her own needs and her adaptation to external reality leads to the development of a false self. Stern (1983), like Winnicott, also associates the negative aspects of the mirroring process with instances of inadequate mirroring. Foulkes (quoted in Zinkin, 1983) explored the possibility of a malignant mirror in the group as reflecting contents the individual cannot contain and thus obstructing the group process and potentially creating a challenging situation for both the conductor and the entire group process.

In Yaron's vignette, the image of the man going down on his knees might have been experienced as a *malignant mirror*, had it been performed cynically instead of empathetically. The playing member's emotional connection to the experience of being desperate that is embedded in this image turned it into a confronting rather than a malignant mirror. If the theatrical response had been performed with cynicism, causing the image to be experienced as malignant, the conductor would have had to examine the source of this cynicism with that particular playing member as well as the entire group later on in the process. The willingness of playing members to live the emotional experience embedded in the images they offer often makes the difference between a confronting yet empathic mirror and a malignant one.

In conclusion, the process of mirroring is a meaningful component of self-development, which encompasses qualities such as validation, containment, reflection, play, empathic presence, observation and disillusionment. This is the foundation for the potentially healing quality of theatrical mirroring. The theatrical response, created in response to the personal story, involves mirroring the story in one or more ways. Theatrical mirroring helps to establish a sense of empathy for and validation of the teller's experience, allowing them to feel connected to the playing members. As seen, mirroring may contain a confronting aspect, which potentially fuels growth and offers motivation to change. Theatrical mirroring works in two directions: the playing members mirror the teller's story back to her and their proposed mirrors influence her; her reactions are then mirrored in the eyes of the playing members. Thus, those mirroring and those mirrored share an experience of mutual engagement and belonging. In this regard, mirroring is a significant therapeutic component, which potentially facilitates development for all group members.

The theatrical mirroring process

The mirroring process begins with the teller sharing a personal story with the group. This can be a memory from the recent or distant past, a moment from their week, thoughts about the future, mixed feelings about some pressing issue in life, a dream, etc. While the story is, in many cases, a personal life story, the teller may sometime choose to tell a story in the third person. Such vicarious stories are perceived through their estimated influence on the teller and their emotional response to it or as a projection from their inner world. In either case, the group members and the conductor listen to the story, collect information and try to identify the story's essence by asking themselves questions such as "if this were a movie, what would it be called?" or "what is this story about?" At the same time, the conductor interviews the teller, asking them similar questions and gathering additional information about the story: its main characters, its unfolding narrative and its central themes. Once the interview is over and after the teller has named his story, playing members respond to the story by presenting a theatrical response. The teller is invited to watch the response – which attempts to mirror his story and inner world – to observe and feel the overt and covert layers of his story.

As mentioned, while the element of theatrical mirroring in Psychotherapeutic Playback Theater mainly relates to the story's overt layer, the theatrical response includes various other layers as well. These include internal voices, feelings, emotions, images, archetypes, reflective aspects and more, which express the more implicit elements of the story and which will be discussed in the following chapters. At this stage, we will focus on theatrical mirroring through three main aspects: (1) the expression of conscious experience; (2) the narrative-formal structure of theatrical response; and (3) dramatic actions.

The expression of conscious experience

The aim guiding the playing members is for the teller to be able to recognize their story in the theatrical response on several different levels: unfolding narrative, content and lived emotional process. Therefore, they seek to resonate conscious emotional and sensory experiences through their mirroring at different points throughout the story's narrative. Accordingly, the echoing of conscious experience takes place at three different levels: the *narrative* level involves acknowledging the teller's narrative, whether by presenting the story's plot (either partially or fully) or by expressing the same narrative structure by means of a parallel story (from literature, mythology, etc.); the *textual* level involves introducing and integrating the teller's own words and phrase into the performance and the *emotional* level involves expressing the teller's overt emotional process. Mirroring at the emotional level is the most crucial because, to a great extent, it determines the teller's emotional reaction to the theatrical response and their capacity to feel understood. Mirroring at the emotional level also determines whether the various perspectives offered by the theatrical response will inspire emotional and cognitive expansion or, alternatively, alienate the teller and lead her to reject them.

In the theatrical response the group presented in response to Yaron's story, one could see the expression of his conscious experience in the playing members' resonance of the teller's overt emotional experience – confusion and helplessness. This was manifest in the very first entrance to the playing space, by the playing member who moved aimlessly in circles. It was further reinforced by the playing members echoing lines from the story such as "I don't know what I'm going to do, everything I do is wrong" or "all I want is for you to be happy."

The significance of expressing the overt emotional experience in the theatrical response is grounded in the thinking of Freud and Klein. In describing his method of dream interpretation, Freud (1900) emphasizes the importance of beginning the interpretation process by asking the dream-teller about the conscious feeling he experienced when waking up from the dream. According to Freud, the expression of this particular feeling is the actual aim of the dream process; as such, it is neither censored nor coded like other dream contents. As a result, the conscious emotional experience of the awake dreamer is an important key to interpreting the dream and understanding his emotional resonance. This enables the interpretation to influence the dreamer on an emotional level, rather than merely on a detached intellectual level. Klein (2002) develops this idea, highlighting the importance of the emotional atmosphere of the dreamer's internalized object-relations. According to Klein, this emotional atmosphere is the first component of one's object-relations that becomes conscious, many times in a senseless manner, and often leads to the development of a symptom. According to Klein, the patient rarely recognizes the repetitive way in which they develop their relationships. For the most part, people seek out therapy as a result of some senseless emotional experience such as unease or an inexplicable sadness or despair. Therefore, the therapeutic process will focus on exploring the nature of the internalized object-relations in which these emotions are grounded. In their descriptions, Freud and Klein view the conscious-yet-unexplained emotional experience as a bridge between the conscious and the unconscious. This bridge plays a crucial role in the patient's emotional resonance during therapy and in shaping the meanings that arise during this process.

Similarly, theatrical mirroring attaches great significance to the expression of the teller's conscious feelings – from the very beginning of the theatrical response. Such direct expression may be illustrated through the musical envelope of the theatrical scene. Without this emotional envelope, we would be left with an intellectual process that is emotionally vacant. While the teller could still take in the various proposed perspectives and the new insights these may give rise to, the lack of basic emotional resonance may lead to *incorporation*. In this state, proposed insights and internalizations "stick in one's throat," without the teller being able to either swallow them or spit them out, to either internalize these newfound understandings or reject them (Klein, 2002).

The narrative and formal structure of theatrical response

This aspect emphasizes the structure of theatrical response in Psychotherapeutic Playback Theater. At the interview stage, the members and the conductor try to examine and identify the essence of the story and the different stages of its narrative. The structure of the theatrical response develops in the playing space in much the same way as conventional theatrical structures and dramatic scene work. In order to provide a mirror that the teller could experience as adapted to their experience and that would facilitate emotional resonance, it is important to offer an aesthetic theatrical piece, which contains the story with its various levels and parts. If, for example, the turning point or the heart of the story is revealed too quickly, this will impair the theatrical aesthetic, undermining the teller's potential for emotional experience. This may result in an incomplete or lacking picture and in theatrical response which does the teller a disservice. We hold that the narrative and formal structure of the theatrical response is psychologically significant, as it creates an aesthetic framework that contains the story and the members' emotional experience. This structure thus encourages the psychological development of all members – the teller, playing members and watching members.

In Psychotherapeutic Playback Theater, three types of structures are commonly used to create a theatrical structure capable of containing the development of the story and its parts: pre-structured theatrical patterns, partially planned improvisations and open improvisations.

Pre-structured theatrical patterns

Theatrical patterns are predefined forms which provide the theatrical response with an aesthetic framework and an organizing container. Their psychic importance lies in their ability to organize emotional experience and provide it with structure and containment. These forms are familiar and known in advance to both the group members and the conductor. Playing members use these to mold the story's contents and its psychological material into a theatrical response with a familiar structure. These theatrical

patterns will be described and examined in further detail in the two chapters dedicated to this subject.

Partially planned improvisations

At the early stages of a Psychotherapeutic Playback Theater group, group
members use partially planned theatrical improvisations. Such preplanning
may draw on the structure of classical Greek tragedy, which allows playing
members to proceed along the story's different milestones: the basic exposition, the introduction of where and when the story takes place, presenting
the characters and their world, exploring their past, offering information
about events that preceded the beginning of the play, giving hints concerning the play's main conflict, presenting the emerging conflict and showing
the characters' actions in relation to the future. This type of minimal, initial
formal outline enables the creation of theatrical response while also expressing the story's various complexions and parts until the theatrical response
reaches its climax and its ensuing resolution. This structure, as an organizing container with boundaries that provide a safe and familiar pre-existing
framework, allows the teller to re-examine his story and reconstruct it,
through the myriad observations offered by the group members.

   In general, every theater piece has two main components – balance and
disturbance: *balance* is a state of equilibrium of different forces, the situation
in which the story's characters existed before the disturbance; *disturbance* is
the sudden emergence of a disruptive factor, which upsets the balance and
creates or releases forces which fuel conflict. Sometimes, the balance is already upset before the piece opens. In every play, there is a character or a
group of characters who upset the balance. When the action representing
the disturbance occurs, the balanced world of the play loses its equilibrium
and begins to change, pushing the plot forward. After a series of actions,
which are the main parts of the piece, the disturbing factor is "defeated" and
balance is restored. This new balance, which is the goal of the play's entire
progression, is different than the one with which the play opened. When improvising, playing members must be aware of these forces, which advance,
inspire and feed the drama, create tension and drive the play's action toward
its resolution.

   To this day, the classical Greek plays remain the most common influence
on theater in general and modern playwriting in particular. The only theater
movement that markedly departs from the values of Greek theater is surrealist theater, which will be discussed in a separate chapter. To introduce the
structure of a partially planned theatrical response, we will briefly elaborate the five main elements of narrative development, as inspired by classical
Greek theater: exposition, dramatic tension, conflict, climax and resolution.

   Exposition – the first stage of the theatrical response is usually some kind
of exposition, which provides the story's basic premise. Its role is to present

the information required for understanding the story. This may include information about the characters and the setting – where and when the plot takes place. The exposition may also hint at the impending conflict, which is the foundation of the story's plot. It is important to present the main question, which serves as the key plotline and upon which secondary questions may be developed, at an early stage in the play. At the same time, we may be presented with opposing sides of the same idea, thereby building dramatic tension. Therapeutically, the exposition provides an opportunity to contextualize and outline the psychological material of the story.

Dramatic Tension – this is the tension created in the audience, which makes them want to know what happens next. The stronger their desire to know, the more they become invested in the plot. Even if the viewer is already familiar with the play's plotline or the story's narrative, they still develop expectations – as they are curious to discover how this familiar material will be portrayed. Dramatic tension encourages members to be more emotionally invested in what is happening in the playing space and results in catharsis when this tension is resolved.

Conflict – this is the intersection where opposing ideas clash. This clash may be expressed through different characters, with each character presenting a different opposing outlook, or through internal conflict, with opposing ideas colliding within the mind of a single character. The most predominate form of internal conflict, appearing in almost every story, is that between the teller's (or the protagonist's) desires and inhibitions. In the classical Greek play, conflict between characters may be expressed through dialogue, while internal conflict may be expressed through a monologue. The conflict may also be between an individual and their destiny or between an individual and society. In all these cases, the conflict raises a problem and the path to resolving it often involves additional conflicts. The way the conflict is played out is often determined by the character's personality. Information about the conflict must be provided piecemeal in order to sustain tension and expectation. The Greek play progresses from one conflict to another, each ending with a small climax and followed by a momentary decrease in tension, a sort of partial resolution. Each subsequent conflict is more difficult and fateful and thus creates more tension, leading up to the play's climax.

While Psychotherapeutic Playback Theater is based on response, the spontaneous and immediate process of theatrical improvisation often utilizes the structure of gradual development toward a core conflict, introduced by the personal story and its ensuing resolution. In this manner, the narrative's theatrical aesthetic is maintained, while engaging both the viewers and the teller. Therapeutically, the conflict plays an important role in fleshing out the contradictory voices in the teller's mind, while providing separate and meaningful solutions for each voice and its distinct needs.

Climax – usually, this is the moment when the play's dramatic tension reaches its peak and the main conflict is presented in its harshest form. The confrontation between the different characters or internal voices becomes extreme, greatly intensifying the central problem. The basic question presented at the beginning of the play, which informed the plot's main arc, now splits off into two opposing world views, presenting each side of the conflict. The height of the conflict also begins to point toward its potential resolution.

Resolution – at this stage, the conflict is resolved or concluded. In classic Greek drama, the resolution may be expressed through the death of the protagonist or even all the main characters. This stage offers some way of solving the conflict expressed in the play. Here, the word "solution" means some kind of change, which transforms the problem, so that it is no longer a burden to the protagonist. In Psychotherapeutic Playback Theater, resolution may involve integration and dialogue between the different sides of the conflict. This type of resolution enables *acceptance* of the different aspects of the teller's experience. The ability to simultaneously contain opposing, even paradoxical, parts creates a complete picture for the teller.

Coda (the final picture) – the resolution is sometimes followed by a coda (final picture). This has various forms and may contain elements of acceptance and resolution, on the one hand, and open up a new question or offer some surprising or revelatory intimation of what is to come, on the other hand. Sometimes, the final picture calls back various elements that were presented throughout the theatrical response.

In his story, Yaron openly expresses the conflict and the distress it involves, creating the need to express these feelings at the very beginning of the theatrical response in order to establish an emotional connection between the teller and the unfolding drama. In order to address this need, the theatrical response skips the exposition and jumps right into the story's conflict – Yaron's wish for his wife to be happy and being helpless and unable to provide her with such happiness in any way known to him. In this case, starting the theatrical response with an exposition and a state of balance might have emotionally alienated the teller to what is going on in the playing space. Instead, the dramatic work heightens the conflict, bringing it to its climax through the language of the playing members' movement and statements such as "do you love me even when I'm not?" and "what kind of husband am I? What kind of man am I?" These statements express and intensify the emotional distress underlying the conflict. Finally, the conflict is resolved through the statement "I need you to trust me. I don't trust myself and I need you to trust me." For Yaron and the other members, this opens the possibility of wanting what is best for the other person, while also containing their feelings of distress. The final picture shows the presence of these different voices together in one playing space – a presence which facilitates their integration and containment in the mind of the teller and the other members.

Fully spontaneous (open) improvisation

After the group has internalized various theatrical, aesthetic and narrative structures, it becomes more capable of producing emotional meaning within a relatively open container, which has a low level of structuring. This allows for open improvisation, which involves no planning or structuring in advance. Once the teller has finished telling his story, members spontaneously enter the playing space, presenting a series of associative images. Even this unstructured setting contains internalized aesthetic and narrative structures which inspire the playing members' theatrical work. Naturally, one such internalized structure is the classical Greek play outlined above. Furthermore, all these structures highlight the stage of theatrical response as both the opening of the theatrical response and an essential condition for its capacity to create emotional dialogue between and within the playing members and the teller. Open improvisation and the structures that inspire it are discussed more extensively in the chapter on different levels of structuring in the theatrical response.

In conclusion, the narrative and formal structure of the partially planned and open theatrical improvisations serves as a container for both the teller and the playing members. For the teller, the structure organizes the narrative and the emotional experience in a way that may imbue them with an unfolding global meaning, which is greater than the sum of its parts, while granting each and every element its own unique place. For the playing members, the structure organizes the improvisation, thus reducing anxiety and uncertainty in a way that may encourage creativity. In addition, this structure is designed to provide inspiration for driving the plot of the response forward, thereby orienting the playing members' mindsets and proposed interpretations.

Dramatic actions

A significant part of the theatrical work process involves the translation of verbal or abstract ideas into concrete theatrical mirroring actions. The teller's story is purely verbal and the theatrical piece transforms it into something tangible through dramatic action. The theatrical mirroring comprises sequences of actions performed by the playing members in the playing space. Each sequence of actions is structured so that each action drives the subsequent action in a manner that allows the entire theatrical response to highlight the links between the different actions. In addition, these actions can also be seen as a means of restoring the balance of the plot. In Psychotherapeutic Playback Theater, each dramatic action expresses an element of the teller's story. For example, when a teller talks about feelings of love toward his spouse, the playing members will translate this into different actions, poses or gestures – such as kneeling, an enamored stare, wooing mannerisms or any other gesture that captures the teller's experience. A single action can express that which many words cannot (Moreno, 1985). For example, walking aimlessly in circles in the playing space made the feelings of confusion and distress in Yaron's story manifest in a vivid and tangible way. The act of kneeling and the relative positions of the playing members in the playing space manifested and heightened the conflict, the emotional experience and the relations between the various characters and voices. In this way, the entire range of the experience is brought to the playing space. The theatrical response brings the story to life, making it tangible for all group members, and transforming it into a living, "here-and-now" experience.

Back to the teller

After the theatrical response, the conductor turns to the teller and tries to gauge the extent to which it accurately mirrored their experience. This act puts control of the story back into the teller's hands. If the teller feels the theatrical response indeed offered an accurate mirroring of their feelings and experiences, the group can move on to the next stage in the process – *sharing*. At this stage, group members verbally respond to the story and the theatrical response processes by telling stories from their own lives that came to mind as they were playing or watching. Once the sharing is over, the conductor recapitulates the various materials that came up and tries to identify a *red thread* – a single theme which is common to all the stories that were shared.

However, if the teller feels that the theatrical response did not approximate their original experience, the conductor is advised to discuss this feeling with them and ask certain clarifying questions, such as:

*   What was missing in the response?
*   What would you have liked to see in the response?
*   If you could extend a part of the response that accurately expressed your experience, which part would you choose?

It is important to understand that the way the teller perceives the theatrical response is subjective and often expresses transference processes. Through this testimony, the conductor and the other group members attempt to understand the process from the teller's perspective. When the teller experiences the theatrical response as too distant from his personal experience, this is an opportunity to examine things more closely, a chance to investigate and go deeper. This is also an opportunity for the teller to use the fact that they are sharing their experience with others to clarify the true nature of their experience. At this stage, the conductor and the other members should try to be empathic and strive to express the teller's experience as accurately as possible in the theatrical response. This approach enables the teller to undergo an important self-reflective learning process, by listening to and observing the different voices that come up in the encounter between their story and the other members, and then mapping which voices were closer to and more distant from their experience and perspective.

It is important to mention that even when the theatrical response is felt to be distant from the teller's personal experience, this still offers an important contribution to the process they and the other members undergo in their encounter with the story. This process contains the therapeutic qualities of *mirroring*, in addition to the elements of validation, growth-promoting and enlightening empathic presence and playfulness. These qualities make it possible to examine alternatives in a safe and playful space.

The therapeutic aspects of this process of specifying the teller's experience in relation to the theatrical mirroring are expressed in Kohut's (1971) notion of *transmuting internalization*. This concept refers to the possible development of beneficial psychological functions within the individual, as a result of *empathic failures* – situations in which their environment failed to react with empathy toward them. These situations allow the individual to restate themselves in a situation which is less of a monologue and more of a dialogue with their surrounding environment. This develops the individual's reflective functions, helping them better explain themselves to themselves and others as well as expanding their experience through internal and external dialogue rather than a blind expectation for compatibility from either their environment or themselves. The transition from empathic failure to the potential emergence of transmuting internalization depends on how the empathic failure is treated. It is important to identify and recognize the distance between how a given experience was experienced by the individual and how it was perceived by others, rather than simply force the observer's perspective on the individual. The dialogue between the two parties should continually strive toward deeper understanding, as this is the basis for the process of transmuting internalization (Osterweil, 1995). In this way, the individual can also feel the concern manifest in the mutual effort to communicate and maintain the dialogue, especially against the backdrop of an experience of difference and separateness (Winnicott, 2009).

In a group for people over the age of 65, held at a retirement home, Arik, a 79-year-old man, talks about how much he misses his wife, who had died eight years before. When the conductor asked which moments he missed the most, Arik replied: "I miss the evenings we spent sitting on the couch together." In response to his story, two members entered the playing space, sat down next to each other and started making small talk: "how are you?" "what would you like for dinner?" "how was work?" This conversation lasted several minutes and, after it was over, Arik said: "that's not it. It didn't look like that." The conductor suggested that he correct the theatrical response and make it more accurate. Arik explained: "just sit next to each other. *You* will be my wife, just put your head on her shoulder and *you* stroke her hair. You don't need to say anything. Just be together." The playing members continued the theatrical response silently, following Arik's instructions. This silent image conveyed the couple's experience of intimacy in a concise manner and both the group members and Arik were very moved. Arik found it difficult to speak and simply said "thank you" with tears in his eyes. In this instance, one could see that the playing members' empathic failure stemmed from their difficulty in containing the emotional overload embedded in this silent and condensed image of intimacy and longing for intimacy. This difficulty was manifest in their choice to make the scene more banal by turning it to an everyday chat, which diffused and dispersed its emotional significance. Arik's correction allowed the playing members and the entire group to contain the emotional experience of intimacy and longing for intimacy. The ensuing group conversation and the following stories highlighted the conflict between containing the experience of longing and the emotional distress it gives rise to and forgetting and dismissing the emotion, in a way that offers immediate relief for the grief one feels when confronted with loss, but leaves one feeling empty.

On a group level, this process is of the utmost importance, as it highlights the group members' subjectivity and differences, facilitating discussion and, in turn, growth. At the beginning of the therapeutic process, group members often hold a view of the group that is laden with projections, split and fragmentary: the group is experienced as a single unit, which is either fully understanding, empathic and accepting, without the need for dialogue, or, on the other side of the split, as completely disappointing, hostile and apathetic. This process facilitates a more integrative view of the group, as containing different voices that one must engage in dialogue in order to achieve true intimacy. Such dialogue is, in fact, the key to growth in the group process (Schlapobersky, 2016).

In conclusion, this chapter discussed the overt levels of the story and ways in which group members mirror these in the theatrical response. Theatrical mirroring has singular therapeutic qualities, validating the teller's subjective experience and thereby providing the foundation for expanding the story and discovering its deeper layers. This may help create new insights and meanings, as discussed in the next chapters. Below, we propose several exercises that emphasize the idea of theatrical mirroring.

Two warm-up exercises implementing the idea of theatrical mirroring

Movement circle

This exercise requires background music, preferably music that expresses many emotional shades, so it could serve as a container for the different voices arising in the group. The first member starts moving in a way that reflects how they are feeling that day, while the entire circle echoes and mirrors their movement. After some 30 seconds, they pass the lead on to another member, who presents their own movement, until all members have had their turn leading the group. Another way of changing the group leader is through spontaneous initiation, in which any member can start a new movement and thereby become the new leader, without being given that role formally. The choice between these two options depends on the conductor's goal: the first method emphasizes the element of correspondence in theatrical mirroring, while the second emphasizes the element of dialogue.

Story analysis

The group is divided into groups of three: one member is the teller and the other two listen and write down their answers regarding the teller's story. They answer three questions –

This is a story about... – in order to identify the story's key motifs, the listeners must try to understand what the story is about and what its main subject is. Completing the sentence "this is a story about..." helps clarify its specific qualities. For example, "this is a story about loneliness; this is a story about hope; this is a story about finding one's way; this is a story about overcoming obstacles." One can also think about the story as if it were a film and try to come up with a suitable title, or offer a title for a single image from the story. While each story naturally has many possible titles, members must pick one to focus on as the core inspiration for the theatrical response.

What is the central emotion of the chosen character? – This question invites members to try and define the overt and clear emotions they recognize in the story.

What is the action of the chosen character? – Members are invited to choose which action in the story is the character's main action, reflecting the story's central elements and inspiring the theatrical response.

The final stage of this exercise is *presenting the story*. After the listeners have answered the three questions in writing, their answers serve as raw material for theatrical work. One of the two presents a monologue in the role of the teller's character (the protagonist) and the other presents a monologue in the role of another character in the story (the antagonist). Next, both characters meet and allow something new to emerge: a dance, a struggle, a conversation or any other type of encounter. Once the theatrical response is over, the teller shares their experience.

Chapter 3

A bypass to the depths of the psyche

Ronen Kowalsky, Nir Raz, Shoshi Keisari

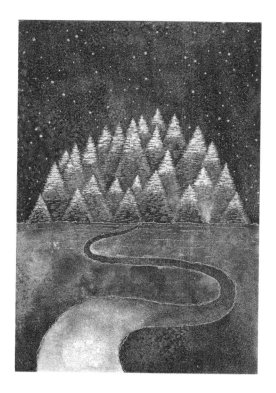

Figure 3.1

In Psychotherapeutic Playback Theater, the personal story encounters the playing space, allowing the group to enter the space of dramatic reality. This space, which exists between reality and fantasy, allows the individual to explore a subjective experience in the "here and now" and creates a free and flexible movement among past, present and future as well as among

DOI: 10.4324/9781003167822-4

different spaces and places (Pendzik, 2006). Jacob Levi Moreno (1965) coined the term "surplus reality," which makes manifest certain invisible aspects of experience. This enables the tangible exploration of aspects that are left unexpressed in our daily reality, such as inner voices, new perspectives that were not voiced in the original story, monologues by inanimate objects that witnessed the events, a conversation with god or a dialogue with people who had died. These aspects can be expressed through a variety of means, including music, movement, theatrical aesthetics and more. In addition, working in the space of dramatic reality allows one to maintain an aesthetic distance from experience, in a manner that produces the kind of perspective that is unavailable in everyday life. This enables the teller to observe their experience at a distance, from the position of a witness (Landy, 2006).

Yuval, a 46-year-old man, shared his difficulty with feeling joy in recent years, ever since his father passed away. He told the group that, whenever he attended a joyful occasion, the memory of his father resurfaced, filling him with sadness and guilt. It eventually became clear that his father had died of cancer and had actually spent his last moments on earth alone, while Yuval was delayed on his way to the hospital, unaware that his father is about to pass away. The conductor asked Yuval to describe his father and their relationship over the years. Yuval depicted a man who was full of vitality and had a great sense of humor, with whom he shared many meaningful experiences while traveling the world together. In the theatrical resonance, one of the members played the role of the teller and another member played his father. With the help of the other group members, the two set out on a shared journey through different places around the world – they strolled down the Champs-Elysees and had croissant and coffee at a local café; they attended an opera together in Milan; they sailed on a gondola in Venice. Then, the character of the cancer made its entrance and the two of them fought it bravely, turning the gondola's oars into swords. At some point, the father froze the scene and told his son that, from this moment on, the father had to continue his journey by himself. He added that he was taking with him, on this journey, all the beautiful moments they shared and asked his son to keep going on these lovely trips around the world, now with his own children. Yuval thanked his father for all the experiences they shared, for the many memories he had of these and for everything his father had given him over the years. Within the theatrical response, a moment of goodbye was made possible, with the two players facing each other, looking in each other's eyes. At last, the two embraced and each went his separate way on the group stage.

Yuval was very moved during the theatrical resonance, attesting that, for him, this was a chance to be present while saying goodbye to his father, something he had not been able to do in real life. The portrayed recollections facilitated the holding of the best moments they had spent together and Yuval noted that this may be a better way for him to say goodbye: holding on to an image of his father when he was healthy, during vital and shared moments, rather than the image of him on his hospital death bed. The theatrical response introduced the possibility that his father had not died alone, but was enveloped by their shared memories and the legacy he left behind: freeing his son to enjoy life with his own children.

Winnicott (1971) called this space "transitional space" – a space that exists in the intermediate area between self and other, fantasy and reality. This area exists in Psychotherapeutic Playback Theater on two levels simultaneously: first, on the level of the encounter between the internal world, as it is manifest in the story, and the external one, embodied by the other members, who function as a "real Other" that is not part of the teller's inner world; the second level is that of the encounter taking place within the theatrical response, bringing together the fantasies and ideas of different members, who function as "real Others" for each other. For example, in Psychotherapeutic Playback Theater, it is possible for one member to offer a metaphoric representation of fantasy, while another member expresses a concrete idea representing reality. This creates an unmediated encounter between the worlds of the self and the other, fantasy and reality, unfolding a new kind of space for the members.

The use of puppets also allows for pronounced expression of transitional space. The process of drama therapy in general and Psychotherapeutic Playback Theater in particular involves a keen awareness of the puppet's significance as both a concrete and tangible inanimate object and, at the same time, a representation imbued with emotional investment (e.g., as "my little sister" or "the new baby"). This sets in motion projective processes that serve as a space for exploring the inner world. Similarly, in Psychotherapeutic Playback Theater, group members function as transitional objects of sorts for one another. It is the Other who is playing a character from the teller's inner world, simultaneously serving as an internal representation and an external Other. This simultaneity establishes and heightens the potential for action in transitional spaces within the group process and, eventually, outside of it as well.

The encounter between the inner world and reality is constantly taking place in theater as well as art in general. The encounter between the abstract idea, the fantasy and reality, embodied by the concrete qualities of the different materials and accessories used (such as the set, the props, the lighting and, most of all, the encounter with the other players), brings forth the potential for transitional space and creativity. This encounter facilitates change and the creation of new meaning. Winnicott describes certain situations in which the encounter between fantasy and reality is made possible, leading to a creative process. In contrast, he also depicts situations in which such an encounter is precluded, because reality is experienced as invasive and destructive vis-à-vis the inner world. In such situations, the person might retreat into excessive emotional investment of fantasy, which is increasingly moving away from reality, and experience its (only) partial realization as intolerable (Winnicott, 1971). Alternately, the person might retreat toward reality, by suffocating their inner world and developing a false self (Winnicott, 1965).

The notion of theater as a collaborative creation turns it into a field of action that is realized in transitional space, creating a dialogue between reality and fantasy, Self and Other. This encounter, which allows a group of individuals to improvise together and explore various ideas in the space of dramatic reality, leads to a more tangible, whole, rich and full expression of fantasy, allowing members to cope with the inevitably partial nature of any realization of fantasy in reality.

For many of us, the term "fantasy" is associated with ideal spaces, wishes and dreams. It should be noted that the fantastic aspects introduced into the space of dramatic reality in Psychotherapeutic Playback Theater are diverse, representing different aspects of the inner world – wants, desires and yearnings, alongside darker parts of the psyche, such as fears, nightmares and aggression. The inner world comprises early memories, various figures, object relations, subjective observations of both positive and difficult events, efficient or distorted interpretations and thinking patterns, wounds and scars, impingements, strengths and coping resources. All these can be explored in dramatic reality. Thus, Psychotherapeutic Playback Theater creates a bypass to the depths of the psyche. The very creation of such a path is a significant milestone in restoring the individual and group capacity to generate dream-thoughts, which in turn support the ability to work through and cope with difficult psychic material (Ogden, 2004).[1]

In Psychotherapeutic Playback Theater, the goal is to express and engage in communication with one's inner parts that is as direct as possible. Such communication, which seeks to bypass the barriers of conscious thought, utilizes the language of dreams, which is based on the use of symbols, images and metaphors as motifs. By simultaneously belonging to two distinct fields of meaning, the metaphor is a manifestation of opposites (Jung, 1964) and serves as a bridge between rational and conscious processes, on the one hand, and emotional experiences and unconscious processes, on the other (Ayalon, 1993 in Lahad, 2006). Improvised theatrical creation constitutes an encounter with a transitional space, which embodies psychic elements much like the language of dreams. It thus facilitates direct communication with one's inner world. The unfolding creation contains images, metaphors and dream-segments, thus paving a bypass that leads directly into the inner world and speaks its language.

Yonit, a 39-year-old woman, shared with the group her deliberation about undergoing fertility treatments and becoming a single parent. Yonit expressed a profound desire to be a mother: she has been feeling this desire for many years, but has yet to find the suitable partner. She is now approaching

40 and she feels that this is her last chance to make her wish of being a mother come true. Nevertheless, she is experiencing a lot of fear about the possibility of being a single mother and giving up her dream of a "perfect" nuclear family, in which mother, father and child share a home. In the reflection, three members entered the playing space, all assuming the role of the unborn child. They got up on chairs and looked down. The first "baby" said: "You should have me. We'll stroll in the park together and you'll change my diapers. You could tell me stories." The second baby said: "Don't give up on me. I must be born. I will bring so much excitement and joy into your life." The third baby said: "God, how much longer can I stay in this waiting room? It's time already! I can't wait for them to call out my name over the PA, so that I could meet you already." After this reflection, the teller said that, at first, she felt disappointed that the group did not show some of her fear of ending up alone. However, as the resonance progressed and the presence of the baby became more tangible for her, she no longer needed that. She felt that the object of her desire was being palpably validated, without any reservation and without the position that held her inner critic. In addition, Yonit shared that the theatrical response embodied the experience of being a family, in which she was together with her baby and was not alone anymore.

Psychotherapeutic Playback Theater entails elements of theatrical aesthetics, which create an aesthetic container for the story. This container enables the reorganization of emotional contents, in a manner that facilitates their reinternalization and their psychic elaboration. It is a reformulation which, much like the language of dreams, allows the observer to experience what happened to them in a surreal fashion and engage in a renewed dialogue with it. The Renaissance period, symbolizing the rebirth of classical ideas in the fields of philosophy, architecture and art, aimed at leaving a profound impression on the spectators, in order to allow them to attain a powerful emotional experience through aesthetic means. Similarly, Psychotherapeutic Playback Theater utilizes the combination of classic theatrical structures that have been revivified and surrealist aesthetics. This combination creates a dual-layered platform, in which surrealist aesthetics corresponds to the primary language of the group members' inner world, while classical theatrical structures provide these contents with a container and a form. This leads to the creation of a meaningful and transformative emotional experience, which is not subjected to conscious realistic logic.

The philosophers and artists of the Renaissance sought to revive the ideas of classical Greece, such as those of Socrates, Plato and Aristotle. In the realm of theater, Aristotle's *Poetics* (2013) was rediscovered. This seminal essay is an attempt to understand the psychic processes undergone by theater spectators, in order to explore which characteristics can make a play a true "poetic" work – one which offers the audience a cathartic and transformative emotional experience. The purpose of the text is to help playwrights strike the most emotional chords of their spectators, providing them with food for thought about their lives (Aristotle, 2013; Zoran, 2009). Aristotle's *Poetics* has inspired key psychoanalytic ideas in theoreticians such as Freud and Jung, aiding their understanding of individual and social psychic processes (Nadler, 1999), in a manner that is still very relevant today.

Psychotherapeutic Playback Theater draws significantly on ideas presented in Aristotle's *Poetics* and their psychoanalytic elaborations. These ideas serve the formation of aesthetic structures capable of containing the various aspects of the story – concrete and realistic representations alongside extrinsic and expansive perspectives, thoughts, feelings and emotions arising from the story and the group. These structures are designed to find a way to bypass rational thinking and lead directly into the inner world, in order to empower the psyche's strengths and facilitate change and development. In addition to theatrical patterns, which are discussed at length in two designated chapters, there are three key concepts in Psychotherapeutic Playback Theater that help create this bypass of conscious experience that produces a profound encounter with one's inner world: (a) expressing attendant feelings; (b) distancing and expansion; (c) fully spontaneous improvisation; (d) nonverbal movement.

Expression of attendant feelings

The attendant feeling is the emotional air expressed in the story. Its significance lies in the fact that it is the opening, the very first element that surfaces in the teller's conscious experience. The attendant feeling serves as a link connecting the teller and the theatrical response. One could liken it to the music that plays at the beginning of theatrical scene work, indicating the emotional ambience even before the scene itself has begun (Fairbairn, 1954; Kernberg, 1995). It is a necessary element, without which theatrical response is experienced as an intellectual and emotionally detached endeavor. The expression of the attendant feeling allows the teller to feel that the other group members understand them, which helps them open up to the possibility of internalizing additional perspectives and expanding their insights into the story. In order to facilitate the emotional expression of the teller's inner world and to define the attendant feeling, the conductor may ask them about the sensory-emotional components of the story and focus on the emotional tone they are immersed in (e.g., "I am feeling ill-at-ease," "an unexplained sadness," "sitting here with a lump in my throat"). The emotional experience is often felt at the sensory-bodily level in a very clear – yet unexplained – manner. Sometimes, the difficulty in feeling an emotion one does not understand results in them telling a story that rationalizes the feeling and ostensibly explains it. It is important to distinguish this rationalization from the raw feeling, which is the key to understanding the hidden layers of the story and of the teller's psyche, as well as to creating the connection between the teller and the other group members.

In fact, the attendant feeling is the emotional exposition of the theatrical reflection and it is crucially important in terms of the latter's emotional impact. Therefore, the very first element of the theatrical response must express the explicit emotion of the story (the attendant feeling). The means for doing so are movement, working with fabrics, playing a character that represents this feeling, using specific theatrical patterns and more. The attendant feeling thus creates the background, the psychic stage set. On this substrate, the characters, relationships, inner and concrete voices, images, possible meanings, perspectives and any other element introduced into the theatrical response can grow, develop and change. The use of musical accompaniment for the theatrical response holds a special significance for the expression of the attendant feeling. Music envelops the theatrical scene and the group members in a sensory-emotional envelope, bypassing the more cognitive verbal parts and opening a direct channel of communication between the preverbal experiences of the different members (Salas, 1993). Therefore, the choice of music is very important and may also serve the conductor as an intervention, seeing that it constitutes a containing envelope for the playing space and the theatrical response.

Julia, a 36-year-old woman, shared with the group an experience of weariness and tiredness that has been part of her life recently. She said that, most of the time, she feels that she is leading a full and fulfilling life, but her extended stay in the big city feels cramped and overloaded. Julia shared that there are moments in which she wants to go back to being a child, to the agricultural community where she was born and raised. She described the open spaces of the fields: "you could spend an entire day walking through them, watching how morning turns to noon and noon turns to night." She talked about the feeling of walking barefoot through fields of grain and how wheat stalks had a particular way of caressing her body and her legs. The group began its resonance with the harmonica solo from the opening of Bruce Springsteen's song *The River* – a piece of music that holds the spacious feeling of open fields, stretching out to the horizon. This musical piece moved the other members deeply and each of them, in turn, came on stage and very vividly shared sensory childhood memories of moments of tranquility and merging with one's environment – "sitting around staring for hours on end, waiting for the sun to set," "feeling the warm sand envelop me with the sound of the waves in the background," "I run with my kite through the open field and suddenly feel a gust of wind catching it and lifting it up, I keep unspooling the string and it flies higher and higher, spinning in the sky." Once the resonance ended, the teller talked about the musical opening and the sensory experiences they shared:

> I suddenly felt my breathing change. You brought this feeling of vast endless spaces, which I was missing so badly and it made me feel that you understand what I'm talking about, in terms of feeling. It's as if you

were right there with me and you have this profound understanding of how it feels. It was also weird hearing all these experiences now, here, as an adult. Now I really want to hear what experiences each of you had that connected you to this feeling.

In expressing the attendant feeling, one can choose a concrete-emotional reflection with a minimum amount of interpretation, expressing a clear and prominent emotion from the story. One can also go farther, widening the scope of interpretation and presenting emotional elements that were not explicitly manifest in the teller's story. The expression of the attendant feeling through the theatrical response can be seen as a kind of therapeutic intervention. Engaging the attendant feeling gives rise to many questions: in some cases, the story is told with an emotional tone that the other members experience as defensive; in others, the story is told in a light and amusing fashion, while it clearly entails more complex emotional contents. In such cases, one wonders whether to reflect the overt, defensive emotion or begin with the implicit emotion straight away. Another example is when the story contains a relationship between two voices, each with its own distinct attendant feeling (such as accuser and accused, humiliating and humiliated, etc.). In these cases, one must choose which of these two voices should be given center stage.

For the members, coming in contact with various attendant feelings and diverse internal characters often gives rise to challenging questions and may even evoke anxiety, especially when dealing with difficult life stories. This raises questions about how useful the expression of unbearable emotions in the theatrical response is for the teller. It also stirs up guilt about the gaps between the different perspectives and emotional understandings presented by the different members. It is important for the conductor and the group members to contain these questions and leave them open. The anxiety the members are experiencing is also an attendant feeling of the entire creative process, validating the emotional experience arising from the story. Ignoring an anxiety-provoking attendant feeling fails to contain the emotional contents of the story and results in emotional detachment. This might, in turn, lead to the experience that the contents of the story are not contained and are not met with true empathy. These issues will be discussed in greater depth in the following chapters.

Distancing and expansion

In Psychotherapeutic Playback Theater, we translate the stories and attendant feelings of the group members into the language of theater. This theatrical language can be concrete and can offer a realistic presentation of the structure and contents of the story. Thus, the reflecting members will depict the teller's overt narrative and the dramatic reflection will express and communicate with the teller at a conscious level. This process is very valuable because it provides acknowledgment and validation of the teller's personal experience and grants them an opportunity to observe their story from the outside, as a witness-spectator watching a theater piece that reflects one of their meaningful life experiences. This level of theatrical work in Psychotherapeutic Playback Theater was thoroughly discussed in the first two chapters of this book.

Another option for theatrical work involves distancing the story to the universal realm of imagination and metaphor. When such distancing of the story is utilized, it is important to try and communicate with the inner world embodied in the story, while maintaining its narrative sequence. Distancing transposes the narrative onto a parallel universe that uses imagery, archetypes and metaphors alongside fairytales, stories from scripture, historical events and more. Thus, for example, if the theme of the story is mother's cooking, this could be distanced to a scene taking place at a restaurant, where one has to pick different dishes. The players could explore what each dish symbolizes, what associations it evokes, how it feels to wait for it to come out, to finally have it served, to take the first bite, etc. Such a scene may elicit a sensual experience involving smells, characteristic sounds and music, emotionally evocative visual forms and cultural or communal associations to the shared story, which carry their own sensory and emotional experiences.

Distancing allows for indirect processing of psychic material and this is one of its prominent advantages. The distance created from one's personal experience is an aesthetic distance (Landy, 1996) and it allows the teller to step back from the immediate emotional content and diminish the emotional charge, which gives rise to defenses. Aesthetic distance thus provides a safe space for observing and exploring one's personal experience. In the above example, it is safer and more comfortable to watch a piece of theater about the emotional representations evoked by various dishes at a restaurant than the emotional representations involving the complex parent-child relationship, as it is manifest through food. The use of distancing should be adapted to the needs of the teller and the group and to the contents of the story. The theatrical response will first include elements of theatrical reflection and then integrate further layers through images, metaphors and distancing.

When distancing is used in theatrical work, the role of the conductor is to make sure that the playing members are working at a level of distancing that is suited to the subjective experience of the teller, the needs of the group and the contents of the story. In this context, it is important for the conductor to keep in mind two states of distancing which are maladapted to the needs of the therapeutic process: over-distancing and under-distancing. Over-distancing occurs when the theater piece includes contents, images and symbols that are too far removed from the contents of the personal story, to the extent that the teller no longer recognizes their own experience in it. This may emotionally sterilize the process, making it a strictly intellectual endeavor. In under-distancing, theatrical work takes place in a space that is far too close to the teller's personal material, emotionally overwhelming them in a way that leads to neither relief nor insight (Landy, 1996). Another way of using distancing in Psychotherapeutic Playback Theater is as a catalyst to the sequence of group associations toward a collective meaning.

In the therapeutic process, *working with a story as a catalyst for a sequence of associations* is a means designed to stimulate group members and lead them to deal with emotional themes and situations in a way that employs aesthetic distance to bypass their defenses. The use of myths, fairytales and healing stories creates an environment that is easy to surrender to while listening, facilitating the listener's connection to the story's protagonist, who is in the process of searching for their identity and sense of self. The story transports the listener to another dimension, one in which images and metaphors are animating and evocative factors (Shtadler, 2017). Myths contain archetypes that are imbued with ancient and universal knowledge about the world as well as various aspects of the collective unconscious, thus offering a bridge to the unconscious (Jung, 1964).

To demonstrate this, we will now present a session that revolved around the Book of Ruth, which emphasizes the stories of two women – Ruth and Orpah. These two women are both Moabites whose husbands had died. While Ruth decides to join her mother-in-law Naomi in the land of Israel and live as a stranger in a strange land, Orpah chooses to remain in her homeland, with her family and part ways with Naomi and Ruth. The session addressed parts of their story, loosely moving between places and events. Even in places where the biblical text provided no information about Orpah's situation, the members themselves were able, by creating an imaginary encounter between the two women some ten years after they went their separate ways, to draw on their own worlds in telling the story of Orpah from their perspective. The members shifted between playing Ruth and playing Orpah, while some chose to play other characters from the book – Naomi, Boaz, Elimelech (the head of the family), Mahlon and Chilion (Naomi's children who died of sickness).

The freedom to move between the various spaces of the story and the ability to choose from among the different roles created an encounter with the diverse materials this story gave rise to as well as with the members' inner world. Next, the members shared personal stories that emerged through their encounter with the story. The group then worked with a personal story shared by Yael, a 45-year-old woman who came back to Israel three years earlier, after having lived several years in the United States. Her family relocated after her husband was offered a job, but Yael shared that, in many ways, she chose to move because she wanted to live abroad and get away from Israel and from her family. During their stay in the United States,

Yael's mother fell ill and Yael faced the painful challenge of being so far away from her, while wanting to be right by her side. She made numerous trips to Israel during this time, but, as a mother of small children who stayed behind in the United States, she was unable to stay away for too long and attend to her mother as much as she would have wanted. When her mother passed away, Yael and her husband decided to move back to Israel so that they could live next to their remaining parents and the extended family. In the therapeutic process, Yael wished to re-process the passing away of her mother, which was saturated with a feeling of pain and missed opportunities given the geographical distance between them. At the group level, the story raised questions that corresponded to the group process and its develop-mental stage – toward the end of the individuation stage and transitioning into the mutuality stage. The story of Ruth the Moabite lent itself to engag-ing themes of surrender versus separation, giving rise to various questions: Are the members willing to be involved in the group process? What does such involvement entail? What does one need to give up in order to feel the safety and mutuality of the group? How long will the feeling of strangeness persist? What can allow more robust feelings of familiarity and belonging?

It should be noted that, much like any other material introduced by the therapist, the story chosen for the group to work on is indicative of the therapist's inner world and contains a statement they are addressing to the group. This means that the choice of text in the therapeutic setting requires considerable reflection. A chosen story might be experienced as an empathic failure: as an interpretation offered by the therapist, which falls wide of the mark of the group's feelings or is introduced too soon, thus exposing the group to something it is not yet ready to face. The role of the conductor is to offer a story that will allow the kind of work that is neither too close to nor too far from the theme the group is engaged in, nothing too schematic, transparent or leading. The introduction of a story that is adapted to the group may be experienced as akin to the therapist's reverie, which offers containment for the members and brings to the surface issues that have yet to be processed or digested (Shtadler, 2017).

Fully spontaneous (open) improvisation

In Psychotherapeutic Playback Theater, members are often encouraged to enter the playing space without any pre-existing ideas, to be "actors who explore on stage," to dance without knowing, to allow a degree of improvi-sation that is as great as possible in relation to the material being evoked in the playing member's psyche and in their interaction with other members. This invitation enables a space that is full of opportunities for listening, ex-ploration and an intuitive creation that is connected to the "here and now." This approach is based on deep listening processes and the felt emotional connection of the members to the contents of the story. Next, the playing members allow spontaneous processes to guide their improvisation through this initial intuitive connection to the story.

This form of work in Psychotherapeutic Playback Theater is called *fully spontaneous (Open) improvisation* (Caines & Heble, 2015). In this mode, the playing member seeks to enter the playing space "empty," "without memory or desire" (Bion, 1967), without any pre-existing knowledge or assumptions, without a personal goal, without planning or any pre-conceived ideas. This type of work involves the crucial element of exploration within the theatrical response. This mode invites a work that is intuitive, much like free associations or "free floating attention." *Free floating attention* is a concept coined by Freud (1912) to depict the kind of listening required by the therapist: a listening which is not motivated by a certain agenda or a search for particular contents, but receptive to the patient's emotional experience, whatever it may be. A position of free floating attention allows the therapist to "listen openly" and take in unconscious material. It is antithetical to the kind of listening aimed at noticing specific contents or subjects, which thereby blocks intuitive and accurate reception of unconscious material. According to Freud (1912), free floating attention is the best method for coming in contact with the patient's emotional experience. Similar depictions that may inspire the playing member to enter this state of attentiveness are also found in Jung's writings (1964). Jung discusses the therapist's associative, dreamlike listening, which supports amplification – the elaboration of the potential meaning of the patient's material – in both therapist and patient.

Working with "emptiness" is likewise important for the process undergone by the playing members. The ability to take in, contain and work creatively and spontaneously within the interpersonal process is one of the cornerstones of the process that allows members to grow through their interaction, to internalize and establish intimate relationships with others. This ability allows members to move forward in a process Bion termed "becoming O" (1984): the ability to face something as is, to contain it within the observer's mind, to learn and grow from one's experience. The fact that theatrical response draws on the material of the Other also makes it a bypassing path for coming in more direct and accessible contact with the inner world of the other members, thus promoting flexibility and receptiveness to one's environment.

Working with "emptiness" often gives rise to reflections about the creative processes themselves as well as to vague emotions, which first appear unrelated to the story's contents. Members often react to these by wanting to expel these invasive thoughts and seemingly irrelevant, even idiosyncratic, emotions. Sometimes, a member will choose not to enter the playing space, because they feel they have no creative ideas. In such cases, the conductor may encourage members to use this feeling of "being stuck" as material to be explored within the theatrical response. It is important to stress that this, in itself, is often highly meaningful material, which reveals profound and significant layers of the inner worlds of all group members and of the emotional processes taking place between them. In fact, these processes are a crucial level of the therapeutic process – the level of inter-personal relations in the group and with the conductor, a level affected by transference, counter-transference and projective identification (Ogden, 1979). It is a level on which unconscious material is transmitted nonverbally between members, in a manner that is felt, but difficult to makes sense of. The absence of planning ahead allows fully spontaneous improvisation to expose members to these processes in the most profound and comprehensive way. The processes of working by means of projective identification and the group dynamics of interpersonal relations will be discussed more thoroughly in the following chapter.

Nonverbal movement

Psychotherapeutic Playback Theater encourages nonverbal response. Words are our familiar language and, by producing habituated cognitive schemes, they may hinder processes of exploration and creation. As associative as they may be, words often express the more conscious processes of secondary thinking, thus resembling a state of being on "autopilot" and only navigating pre-established paths. The powerful stage presence of words may block creative and exploratory processes which lead to new discoveries. In contrast, movement-based representations provide a broader space for multiple and diverse interpretations. In the playing space, movement-based representations allow the witnessing teller to project material from their inner world, thereby also expressing this material. The more abstract a movement-based representation is, the more it allows for a wider range of interpretation.

Because group members are usually less fluent in the language of movement than they are in verbal language, it is important to facilitate the kind of work that will invite them to explore the language of movement, for example, through the *working with images pattern*. In this pattern, members are divided into groups of three, with one member as a teller and the two others as players. The teller is instructed to share a story that has been on their mind that day. As the teller shares their story, the other two members listen, without reacting or asking any questions. After the teller has finished, they are asked to come up with an image the story has evoked in them. They are instructed not to plan ahead and to use as much movement and as little words as possible.

The first player enters the playing space, uses movement to present the image that emerged in them and then freezes. The second player does the same; they may relate to the sculpture created by the first player (though they do not have to). The resulting shared sculpture is maintained for several seconds. Then, the two images come back to life, side by side, and eventually meet to create a movement-based dialogue. At the end of each response, the three members have a brief sharing circle, recounting their experiences of watching and performing. This entire pattern can be repeated three times, switching roles so that each member can experience the role of teller.

This kind of work allows members to experience a more open improvisation, which is less reliant on pre-existing ideas and thoughts. The members can explore the type of discourse that emerges within and as a result of the kind of work that is more movement-based and intuitive – a discourse that has more room for projection, for the expression of the unconscious interaction between members, for abstraction and for multiple interpretations.

In conclusion, Psychotherapeutic Playback Theater is aimed at facilitating a creative process, which bypasses conscious experience and invites members to deepen and expand their inner world, by revealing additional layers within the story. Relating to the attendant feeling, to processes of distancing and expansion, to intuition and creativity within the improvisation enables a dynamic movement that allows the story to unfold into new dimensions.

Note

1   For its psychodramatic applications, see Ryvko (2005, 2018); for applications in the field of group analysis, see Friedman (2002).

Chapter 4

Opposites and integration

Ronen Kowalsky, Nir Raz, Shoshi Keisari

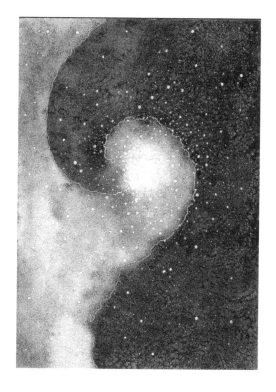

Figure 4.1

In this chapter, we will explore the story, the theatrical response and the group process through the hidden opposites these entail, through the encounter between two voices that creates contrast and conflict. Quite often, the process of identifying the opposing forces in a story serves as a significant gateway for pinpointing the essence of that story and imbuing the theatrical

DOI: 10.4324/9781003167822-5

response with richness and depth, which can promote meaningful reflective processes among group members. This chapter discusses the use of the notion of opposites and conflict as a path for recognizing and embracing more fully various aspects of the teller's experience and their theatrical expression and for moving toward new discoveries and developments.

Personal stories often introduce two sides or aspects, which represent opposing driving forces. In many cases, one of these aspects is clearer, more explicit and externalized, while the other is implicit and requires active uncovering and exploration. The knowledge that there is a certain level of experience which is two-fold and split, containing two opposing sides, may in itself facilitate acknowledgment of those hidden parts of the story and support their movement toward integration.

Thus, for example, when a teller shares a story that features a prominent role with a strong need for control, one would do well to also look for the opposing role, which feels helpless or lacks control. A story which expresses an experience of aggression should give rise to the assumption that it involves an implicit experience of vulnerability. It is important to subsequently portray both these roles in the theatrical response. Once the two sides have been identified, one can further explore and understand each side separately, until a third option becomes available – one that allows for the integration of these two ostensibly contradictory aspects of experience.

The process of Psychotherapeutic Playback Theater is often manifested in a creative search for hidden internal parts. The empathic listening to the story and the desire to benefit the teller lead playing members to use the theatrical response to focus on expressing the explicit parts of the story. However, in order to offer a full experience of the story, one capable of providing a broader perspective, they should also find ways to express opposing voices – voices that were not presented in the explicit story – in order to reveal the complexity of the internal world that drives this story and is manifest in it.

For members to be able to observe both sides of this coin, it is recommended that they apply a technique of *deconstruction and clarification*. In order to take account of the various parts and internal voices featured in the story in a more focused manner, it is vital that one conducts a differentiating analysis of these parts. This is done by deconstructing the story into its distinct voices and exploring each voice separately. This process facilitates the clarification and highlighting of the various elements of the human psyche. Once the different voices have been deconstructed and clarified, one can move on to reconstructing them in the process of creating an integrative image. These processes of deconstruction and reconstruction are conceptually grounded in Melanie Klein's object-relations theory (1975) and Thomas Ogden's later variations on it. In order to understand how these processes take place on the psychic level and how they are manifest in the therapeutic process of Psychotherapeutic Playback Theater, we will present a brief explanation of the two positions conceptualized by Klein (1946) – the paranoid-schizoid position and the depressive position.

The paranoid-schizoid position

In the first months of life, the baby's experiences are formless and comprise phantasies and drives. The paranoid-schizoid position enables a primary way of organizing this experiential chaos by means of two key features: splitting (hence the schizoid part) and persecutory anxiety (hence the paranoid aspect). The role of splitting is to introduce a primary, survival-oriented way of organizing experience through the distinction between good and bad. Klein (1975) used the terms "the good breast" and "the bad breast" to represent the structure of the baby's experience as constituted by two opposing poles: when the baby is sated and satisfied, it feels loved by the good breast; when it is hungry or distressed, it feels persecuted and hated by the bad breast. The attribution of internal hunger and distress to an evil external object grants this position the title of "paranoid." In the experience of splitting, there is no memory; being is absolute and, from the baby's perspective, exists eternally. When the baby is suffering or having difficulties, this experience is absolute and amounts to the notion that "I'm bad, the world is bad, everything is terrible; it always has been and always will be." The baby feels that its momentary experience always existed and will exist forever. Even when the baby has a good experience, which too is experienced as absolute: "I'm good, the world is good and we are one and the same." Here, too, the present experience is felt to be eternal – "it has always been like this and always will be."

   This kind of splitting persists into adulthood at a certain level of experience and internal organization. For example, when falling in love: on one side of the split, the love object is viewed as a perfect person ("he understands me, of course we're going to keep seeing each other, this relationship looks promising") and the various elements of life seems to fall into place reassuringly ("I'm having a perfect day today: all the traffic lights are green. No traffic, the weather is perfect; the radio is playing all my favorite songs. I've finally realized that life is beautiful and worth living. Everything is wonderful and great and is going to stay that way forever"). The other side of the split can come into play, for example, when one experiences rejection ("everything is bad. Everyone is ugly, the world is nasty, and the radio is playing terrible songs. The country is going to hell, politicians are corrupt, there is no future and now I've discovered the truth: things have always been this way and always will be"). Both these experiences color one's entire being, both backward (in retrospect) and forward in time, and are felt to be eternal truths. Furthermore, the negative experience of the split gives rise to the need to find someone to blame. This aspect represents the persecutory anxiety characteristic of the paranoid-schizoid position: someone is responsible for this terrible state of affairs (e.g., "the person who left me is to blame for all this, because he is unworthy of me and wants to harm me"). Another example, taken from the world of groups, is when one member experiences a negative feeling during a session and then projects it onto the other group members ("you're all so condescending"). In all these instances, the negative experience is projected onto the other in its entirety.

Yet another aspect of the paranoid-schizoid position is a lack of differentiation between self and other. The other is not experienced as a subject who has an inner world, a perspective and needs of their own, but as an object that either succeeds or fails in addressing the needs of the self. This is why Klein chose to use the terms "good breast" and "bad breast" instead of "good mother" and "bad mother." This aspect can be demonstrated by a story shared by a woman describing her break-up with her partner. Immediately after she had broken up with him, she tried to seek comfort by calling her friend, but there was no answer. The paranoid-schizoid position entails split patterns of thinking (such as "this friend is not picking up because she's selfish, maybe she's even happy that we broke up"). The thought that this friend may have her own needs that are keeping her from answering the phone at the moment is utterly absent from the teller's range of emotional thinking. There is a sense that the individual and the world are one and the same and the person experiences themselves as being in possession of the truth – in contrast to everyone else. This abolishes the subjectivity of the other; one's experience is absolute and the other is either for or against one, leaving no room for doubt. This position also gives rise to the wish to be understood by the other or the group without the need for dialogue; this wish is significantly present throughout group therapy processes, especially at the beginning.

The depressive position

The baby needs the paranoid-schizoid split in order to organize its experience, but it also has an inherent proclivity for integration. Thus, as it develops, the baby begins to perceive its mother as an object that contains both good and bad aspects and, eventually, comes to view her as a subject in her own right. While this view decreases the level of anxiety caused by the paranoid position, the abolition of the schizoid split leads to the depressive position. This is because the fusion of the good and bad parts of the mother impairs the phantasy about the purely good mother, which now entails certain bad aspects as well. In order to shift from the paranoid-schizoid position to the depressive position, two prerequisites must be met: first, a sufficient level of cognitive development; second, the accumulation of enough good experiences.

As mentioned, the key characteristic of the depressive position is the integration of good and bad. Unlike the paranoid-schizoid position, which divides the world into good people and bad people, the depressive position features all manner of human subjects (each of them possessed of their own life, motives and ideas) as well as a differentiation between self and other. The depressive world has colors and shades, but these are not as intense or contrasted as those of the paranoid-schizoid position. Thus, the adoption of this position is accompanied by the difficult and painful experience of losing the absolute good. Yet another price one must pay is the element of personal responsibility. The person realizes that the world is not necessarily out to get them and that they are responsible for their own life situation. Take, for example, a person who, as a child, viewed his parents as the personification of all that is good and perfect in the world and who believes that a purely good life would be possible for him, if he only followed their example. For this person, the process of maturation and development brings about the insight that his parents had tried to make the best of their lives and that they succeeded in some ways and failed in others. This leads to the discovery that he himself, when he grows up, will try to live his best life and that his life will have certain good aspects, alongside certain difficulties and obstacles.

In Psychotherapeutic Playback Theater, we can utilize the Kleinian positions as milestones in the unfolding theatrical response. During the initial stages of the response, the splitting and the different parts are clearly presented through the deconstruction of the story to its inner voices and the heightening of the contrasts and opposition between these voices. It is important that the teller recognizes the split through which the various voices are expressed in a clear and distinct manner. This is the first stage of the theatrical response, which corresponds to the paranoid-schizoid position. It is important to reach this stage before introducing any reconciliatory or integrative theatrical actions, which correspond to the depressive position. Rushing through this process may lead to premature integration, which might be experienced as a "didactic," externally dictated and moralistic input, designed to silence certain voices or parts.

In many ways, we view conflict and splitting not only as patterns that represent the relations between different intra-psychic forces, but mostly as a structuring intervention that seeks to extract, delineate and flesh out silenced voices. Only after each part has been elucidated can one create a dialogue between the various split parts. This dialogue first allows the teller to see that these voices can co-exist and only later on leads to the emergence of a third, integrated option.

Ronit, a 26-year-old woman, told a story about her complex relationship with her mother. Ronit said that, when she was 16, the two began to drift apart because of her wish to start dating boys, going out with her peers and attending parties. Her mother expressed her essential difficulty in accepting Ronit's choices and lifestyle. Such statements undermined their relationships and made Ronit feel alone and unaccepted by her family. Recently, this difficulty was exacerbated further, when Ronit chose to leave her parents' house and move to Tel Aviv, while still unmarried. As Ronit was telling her story, the conductor asked her to describe her mother and depict her behavior, her life choices and her character. Ronit described her mother as a harsh woman, who grew up in an ultra-orthodox home, in a culture where women are not supposed to engage in intimate relationships before marriage.

To her mother, an intimate encounter with a man could severely hurt Ronit and this thought is unbearable to her. In addition, Ronit depicted her mother as a woman who is very preoccupied with caring for her children, making their needs her first priority and sometimes being overprotective.

Two women players came on stage. One of them reflected Ronit's experience – her wish for freedom and the feeling of being rejected by her mother whenever she is "appalled" by one of Ronit's life choices. The first player represented the voice that said: "I am an adult and I have my own life experience to draw on; I am mindful of the choices I make; trust me and grant me the freedom to live my life." The second player portrayed the mother, presenting her anxiety and the terror that something horrible might happen. This player presented the voice that said:

> I am your mother and I have to keep you safe; you don't know how dangerous it can be out there; I don't want you to crash. I'm here to watch over you and I will do anything to keep you from getting hurt, even if that means you being angry at me. I'm only doing this for your own good.

The position of two such characters side by side on stage enables the splitting of any perspective; when the two voices are expressed within a single theatrical scene, this facilitates integration, without relinquishing the unique character of each distinct voice.

According to Klein (1975), when the loss of the absolute good is too difficult to bear, manic defenses are mobilized. The *manic defense* is directed at one's dependence on the disappointing object ("who needs him, anyway," "forget about him, he's not worth you and your tears"). These processes deny dependence and pain and preclude any encounter with the feelings of heartbreak and pain that accompany loss. The manic defense shifts the person back to the paranoid-schizoid position while, for example, casting the abandoning boyfriend being in the role of absolute evil. According to Klein, the manic defense helps one deal with pain, but it also limits processes of learning and development and reinforces repetition compulsion and the repeating of internalized object-relations constellations, by which the same relationship is reiterated in different variations without the ability to understand the internal motive causing it. This is because manic defense places the person between the position of victim and the position of "the one who aggressively beats the aggressor," but prevents them from assuming responsibility and thereby learning. Klein (1975) suggests that a better way of coping with the loss of absolute good is the wish for reparation. This process involves assuming responsibility over the resulting situation, gaining a deeper understanding of the internal motives for its creation and seeking to change these factors and their reenactment in future relationships. Through reparation, one remains in the depressive position. In contrast, the manic position, which creates imaginary reparation that denies internal motives, causes one to regress to the paranoid-schizoid position.

In Psychotherapeutic Playback Theater, we sometimes see the emergence of manic reparations in the playing space, stemming from the members' sincere wish to help the teller cope and to ease their pain. In many cases, this leads to the opposite result – the teller feels that the group was unable to contain and cope with the complex and painful feelings they shared, and thus had to resort to manic reparation. It is important that the theatrical response succeeds in rendering the pain and loss of the conflict present rather than achieving reparation without confronting and dealing with the difficulty at hand. Common examples for manic reparation can be seen in stories that involve a present difficulty whose theatrical responses strives to attain a "happy ending" at all cost. Members of Psychotherapeutic Playback Theater groups often use the metaphor of "gift giving" to represent their wish to use the theatrical response to give the teller something meaningful – a "gift" that will allow them to grow and discover their inner resources. Despite its ubiquity, we view this metaphor as a potential trap, which diminishes the therapeutic process. This is because group members sometimes interpret this notion of "gift giving" as a need to create a theater piece that has a "happy ending" no matter what; even when such a "happy ending" is inappropriate to the story at hand or when it fails to validate the teller's experience or to contain the feelings of loss and pain expressed in the story, thus limiting the potential for introspection, coping and development. In addition, a forced "happy ending," which is not adapted to the contents of the story, may send the message that the contents of the story and the conflict it entails were too difficult for the playing members to contain or deal with. This situation may leave the teller feeling guilty about introducing material that was too difficult into the group, heightening their sense of isolation and lack of validation.

Ernesto, a man of 35, told the group about a difficult move to a new apartment, which began with his old landlord suddenly informing him that his lease will not be renewed and that Ernesto will be forced to leave the apartment he has been living in for several years, which had been his home throughout significant times in his life. He had very little time to pack up all of his things and move to a new apartment, which was a compromise because of the circumstances and the limited amount of time he had to find a new place to live. His move was fraught with trouble: the movers came late; the new apartment was noisier than he had thought and there were various damages that required additional work – far beyond what he had expected. His overall feeling was one of weariness and dissatisfaction, disappointment and a sense of being uprooted and "homeless." Ernesto described a certain moment at which he sat down on his boxes, looked at the chaos that surrounded him and all the work that still needed doing and was overwhelmed by helplessness and despair.

In response to his story, the group created a theatrical response that reflected the experience of moving apartments, dealing with the suddenness of the move and the heightened activity of all the packing, carrying and setting up. To finish their scene, the players decided to add a "happy end," where everything was neatly in its place and Ernesto was sitting in his new home. He was having friends over to watch an FC Barcelona soccer match, drinking beer and eating snacks, then Lionel Messi scored a goal and everyone jumped up and screamed with joy: "Goaaaaaal." Once the theatrical response was over, the conductor, having noticed this premature and overly positive reparation, asked the players to return to the stage and portray the difficulty, the confusion and the feelings of helplessness and despair arising from the story. In their second response, the theatrical expression of these experiences was performed silently, through the repetitive movement of the players and their facial expressions as they moved boxes back and forth, from one side of the stage to the other. As the reflection progressed, the boxes became heavier and heavier and the players had less and less energy to carry them.

Ernesto commented on the two theatrical responses he had watched. He explained that the first one was positive and made him feel good, but the second one made him feel that the players were deeply and empathically connected to his difficulty and his experience in a manner that was more complete. It was the reflection of his difficulty and despair that allowed him to feel the massive impact this move had had on his life and allowed him to touch on his difficulty with transitions in general and a key theme of his life – being an immigrant and the need to be rooted and anchored.

It should be noted that later developments of Klein's notion of the two positions – such as that offered by Ogden (1992) – highlight the importance of both positions as well as the transition between them. According to Ogden (1992), the ability to split off and explore each internal voice in a distinct manner, as if it were the only one, is also highly significant. Premature integration is forced and false, leading to emotional detachment and the avoidance of one's full emotional experience. Similarly, Ogden also highlights the significance of the *manic defense* as a step on the path toward the wish for reparation. In his view, certain empowering experiences are only available during the stages of manic defense and it is important for these to be experienced and included in the emotional material that will eventually become integrated. Much like Ogden, Jung (1916/2003) also discusses the principle of the union of opposites as a critical divergence from one's process of development and individuation. According to Jung, true development is achieved by understanding and accepting the paradox by which human wholeness involves the containment of opposing forces within a single person.

The use of conflict-based theatrical patterns allows for the explicit exploration and holding of each side of the story. The presence of both sides within a single pattern, even when they are distinctly apart, enables the simultaneous containment of the story's complexity and its main aspects. The next section, therefore, discusses the theatrical expressions that bring together the story's opposing forces.

Objective and obstacle

Two elements which drive the dramatic scene are the objective and the obstacle. Drama is the action which results from the collision between the objective and the obstacle. The objective constitutes the character's emotional investment in whatever it is they seek to attain. In each story or play, the character has a central objective as well as secondary objectives, which vary from scene to scene and according to which character they are addressing. The obstacle constitutes the various factors preventing the protagonist from investing their psychic energy in an activity or an object. It should be noted that the obstacle is not there to stop the character; rather, its presence represents the complexity of the story and the manner in which the different characters are motivated by different and opposing forces. Quite often, the obstacle is manifest in the form of another character or an internal voice in the story. The obstacle of a given story can also be a person's narcissistic vulnerability or their own anxieties and defense mechanisms, which prevent them from attaining objectives which are perceived as harmful.

These two opposing forces are expressed in an extreme and distinct fashion in fairytales. The archetype of the hero in fairytales and myths illustrates the principle of objective and obstacle on a universal level (Jung, 1916/2003; Neumann, 1989). For example, the objective of the warrior hero is to retrieve the healing stone from the kingdom of darkness. This is her destiny: to save her birthplace and put into action her courage, her powers and abilities, her wisdom and accumulated skill. Simply riding her horse there and fetching the stone will not produce any drama in the story. Therefore, the story must have a dragon (an obstacle) whose role is to guard the stone against the hero. The more powerful the dragon, the greater the hero's desire to attain her objective and the greater the drama of the story. In fact, this resonates with the internal psychic structures of the listeners.

Freud (1917) defined the term *cathexis* as a psychic energy which is invested in certain objects (such as significant people, activities or parts of the body) and which is part and parcel of the natural course of development and the need to establish meaningful relationships. Cathexis sustains one's liveliness and creativity and allows one to experience life as satisfactory. Freud called the counterforce, which stops cathexis from being realized, *anti-cathexis*. These terms were borrowed from Aristotle's *Poetics*, in which it is argued that conflictual struggles create drama and make the play a "poetic" one, meaning a play that portrays a profound psychic experience that reflects the various crossroads of life (Nadler, 1999; Zoran, 2009). Following Aristotle, Freud (ibid.) argues that the greater the anti-cathexis, the greater the cathexis; the greater the prohibition, the greater the desire. As the obstacle grows more formidable, so the desire to obtain one's objective or object grows more powerful. A clear example of this can be found in reality television shows, in which the emotional investment in a certain member is increased in relation to the difficulties they endure. This is how, according to Aristotle (2013), a good play presents the audience's most potent hopes and most radical fears.

In Psychotherapeutic Playback Theater, we sometimes use a theatrical pattern that holds two fundamental voices: "objective" and "obstacle." The teller describes an object of desire, something they want to have, as well as the inner voice that is stopping them from consummating this desire. Two players enter the group stage: one expresses the objective while walking toward a certain point in the room, while the other gives voice to the obstacle, while physically trying to stop the first player. In one session, Sandra, a woman of 40, expressed her desire to write a children's book about the learning difficulties from which she suffered her entire life. She expressed her wish to create a book that used images to validate the experience of children with learning difficulties, based on her own personal knowledge and experience as well as decades of clinical work with children with attention deficit/hyperactivity disorders and learning difficulties. The member who played the objective moved through the room, walking to some imaginary point in space and saying:

> this is great, you have accumulated so much knowledge and experience, no one understands better than you the experience of a child who walks through this world with acute ADHD... a book that is full of images will definitely touch these children and help them grow stronger... you can make time for it during the summer and write.

The member who played the obstacle expressed the various voices that weakened her will and her ability to bring her idea to fruition:

> You can't do it... only writers can write books... what are you thinking? Who do you think you are? You'll probably start it and never be able to finish... like so many other things you've tried in your life.

Two roles engaged in a struggle take the stage: one wants to move forward, presenting the voice of motivation, creative passion and faith in one's path, while the other tries to stop it and take the wind out of its sails. This image offered Sandra a clear reflection of her powers and the fact that she is giving too much room to the critical voices that are disempowering her while she is trying to make her dreams come true.

Another theory that can help clarify and explore the different and opposing sides of an experience and present it clearly in the playing space is role theory, one of the approaches of drama therapy.

Role theory in drama therapy

The core of working in dramatic space is the human capacity for playing roles. Moreno (1961), the father of psychodrama, defined the term "role" as the tangible and actual forms of the self through which the individual responds to a certain situation that involves other people or objects. Landy (Landy, 1996; Landy et al., 2003) views the notion of "role" in drama therapy as an assortment of qualities (characteristics, emotions, thoughts, behaviors) that represent a certain aspect of a person (such as the roles of hero, witch or mother). Much like Jung's (Jung, 1916/2003) notion of archetypes, Landy (1996) sees the role as a virtue of unique characteristics and qualities, with different degrees of deviation from those qualities.

The adult individual deals with a broad range of roles in their life, roles that often differ from one another and are sometimes even opposing and contradictory. People tend to try and find a balance between their roles and can tolerate the paradoxes and even conflicts between their various roles. As a construction of one's life story, personal identity allows for the integration of these roles into a single self, with an adequate level of unity and purpose (McAdams, 2001). Theatrical experimentation allows one to explore the roles one plays in life, try out new roles and examine other roles that one has never played before (Landy, 1996; Landy et al., 2003).

Once a story has been introduced into the group space, we begin by identifying its prominent and explicit dramatic roles – the mother, the jester, the hero, etc. These roles represent clear aspects of the teller, which are explicitly presented in the story and which manifest parts of the teller's self. After the *explicit dramatic role* has been identified, one moves on to explore and study it – how it moves through the playing space, how it expresses itself in front of the other characters, the situations in which it comes to the fore – in order to achieve a clear expression of its various qualities. Next, one can move to the following stage, which allows a deeper exploration of one's experience by introducing the counter-role: a role which, in most cases, is not explicitly present in the story, thus necessitating a process of active extrapolation and inquiry.

The *counter-role* represents qualities that are the opposite of those of the explicit role. It is not necessarily an inverse role, even though it is experienced as such in many cases. Rather, it is a role that represents different, more hidden, aspects of the explicit role. For example, Landy (2000) proposes that the role of the mother can be juxtaposed with a set of counter-roles, such as those of father, daughter and brother, or an entirely different role which pertains to the particular story. For instance, if the mother in the story is associated with the experience of being punished, the counter-role can be that of helper, of someone who supports or contains. After the counter-role has surfaced, one can explore it more deeply through movement, text, music and cloth or by creating situations that bring it to life. At this stage, it is important that each role is clearly and distinctly defined and expressed, so that the contrast between the different roles can allow the teller to access a deeper level of experience. The first image is that of the explicit role, while the second image is that of the counter-role, with the two roles being clearly distinguished and even thoroughly split off. Each role exists separately, so that each aspect of the story is explored by itself within the theatrical response. Only after each role has been imbued with a clear voice, which holds its respective aspect of the self, does the third image emerge.

The *third (integrated) image* is an image that creates a dialogue between the two roles, reconciling them in a manner that allows them to co-exist. Landy (ibid.) defined this part of the work as a guide, which allows the two qualities to express themselves simultaneously. Thus, Landy's role theory uncovers the processes of *deconstruction*, in which the story is deconstructed into its constituent roles; *splitting*, in which the contrast between these roles is heightened; *clarification*, in which each role is brought on stage and explored separately; and the *reconstruction* of the story through the act of integration. It is important to note that the process of creating the guide, the integrated image, cannot be fully realized unless it has been preceded by the clarification and exploration of the unique voices associated with each role. After being grounded in this work, the concluding image manifests a more complete and whole integration of the different aspects of the story.

Daniella, an 82-year-old woman, participated in a Psychotherapeutic Playback Theater group at an adult day care center. In one of the sessions, the conductor presented a list of dramatic roles (taken from Landy's "Taxonomy of Roles"; see Landy et al., 2003) and asked the members to choose one role that they recognize in themselves. Daniella chose the role of the "naïve" person. She shared that, up until the age of 40, she was innocent, a devoted wife and mother whose husband and family were her entire world. At 40, she found out that her husband was cheating on her and that everyone around them already knew about it: she was the only one who believed that he loved her. She then put her faith in the attempt to maintain marital harmony and mend the relationship, but today she realizes that she had been too innocent, too naïve. A player came on stage and played the role of the naïve person for Daniella, showing how she walks across the room, what she says: "I am innocent, I am good, and I will do everything to keep marital harmony, to secure the love of my husband and my children." When the conductor asked Daniella to pick a counter-role, she chose that of "warrior." She said that, when she finally came to her senses and realized that her husband had betrayed her trust, she decided to fight him, to make sure that she kept the house for herself and her children. This was a side of herself that she had not known before. Another member took the stage and played the role of "warrior" for her, saying: "I am going to fight him, I'm going to do everything for my children, and I won't let him steal our home from us." Next, the conductor instructed the two roles to engage in a dialogue. The "warrior" said to the "naïve" person: "wake up, come on, rouse yourself, go out and fight! Can't you see what he's done to you?" The naïve person replied: "I'm all about peace and love, I want to keep having Friday night dinners with everyone, to see my family, and I don't have the strength or the energy to fight." This dialogue led to the birth of a new role. Daniella said:

> that's the kind of mother I am; that's the role of "mother." On the one hand, I'm all about peace, solidarity and love, but on the other hand, I'm willing to fight for my home and my children. This is how, at my age, I'm still cooking these huge dinners for everyone, so that we can all come together and fill our home with that Sabbath feeling, each and every Friday.

This example illustrates how the dialogue between opposites gave birth to the integrated role, which is capable of holding both qualities at the same time.

Yet another aspect of structuring the therapeutic process in the playing space that originates in Ogden's theory (1994) concerns different levels of experience organization. Ogden argues that one of the fundamental motivations of human behavior is the avoidance of identification with an expression of certain roles that involve certain emotional experiences. These are experiences which, throughout a person's development, evoked harsh judgment and criticism and are therefore associated with difficult feelings of shame, guilt and anxiety. This may lead to premature integration, which acts as an extension of such avoidance by offering the person a highly diluted taste of the forbidden role and the emotional experience it entails. This state of affairs leads to an emotional experience which, while rational and true to life, has an "after-taste" of emotional impoverishment and emptiness. According to Ogden (ibid.), the full process must include the transition from identification with the person's default role to complete emotional immersion in the forbidden role and the emotional experiences it involves. Only then can true integration of the two roles and experiences be attained and, in turn, facilitate the emergence of new roles and emotional experiences.

Opposite sides – the psychic construction of conflict through theatrical patterns

In Psychotherapeutic Playback Theater, theatrical patterns serve to structure the theatrical response. Each pattern is conducive to a specific psychic process and thus facilitates the attainment of different therapeutic goals, which correspond to different kinds of psychic materials. One should distinguish between using a theatrical pattern as a way of creating a dramatic reflection of the present state of the teller, a kind of mirror image, and using it as a way to deconstruct and reconstruct the story in a manner that facilitates new discoveries and further development for both the teller and the group. In this section, we will present three different theatrical patterns – *back to back*; *one behind the other*; and *cross* – which create different types of relationships between the differentiated sides of the conflict. We will discuss the differences between these theatrical structures that are designed to express conflict and show which types of stories can be expressed dramatically through each pattern.

Back to back

This pattern for working with conflict creates and heightens the clarification of the emotional material presented in the story. It does so by allowing each side of the conflict to voice itself separately. This technique achieves the qualities of focus and elucidation.

The two playing members decide in advance which one of them will play which side of the conflict. It is important to instruct them to speak in the first person. The presentation of the conflict is done as a kind of aside, with each playing member sharing his thoughts with the audience. They explain to the spectators why their position is the correct one and constitutes the absolute truth. If necessary, the polarization of the two views should be increased even further, so as to render each side's standpoint more specific.

Next, the two playing members stand back to back, in profile to the audience. They are instructed to keep revolving around an imaginary axis that is set between them and to complete three such revolutions, while staying back to back. Thus, each member presents their chosen side of the conflict while moving through the semi-circle that faces the audience. When they reach the point where they are once again in profile to the audience, they stop talking and the other member starts presenting their chosen side of the conflict.

This intervention is particularly significant in situations where the teller's inner world gives rise to a jumble of different voices. The acts of deconstruction and clarification gives each voice a chance to be heard without having to fight for its place among all the others. After the teller has heard the various voices, the rotation of the two playing members creates a way for moving between the two voices as well as connecting them internally through aesthetic means. This form corresponds to psychic processes, which are characteristic of the paranoid-schizoid position, in which two distinct experiences or inner voices cannot co-exist side by side. They are thus linked by the teller and the audience, who watch the disjointed parts being simultaneously present in the playing space, with each part as an independent whole.

In Psychotherapeutic Playback Theater, the opposing sides should be brought to light theatrically, in clear and distinct manner, so that each player is completely loyal to the side they are portraying and refrains from expressing elements associated with the opposing viewpoint. This is an intricate action that members often experience as unnatural, seeing as they often tend to try and express in the playing space the entire range of voices that have come up in the story. This stems from a wish to express the teller's confusion and the feeling of uncertainty arising from the conflict as well as to present an experience of reconciliation or false reparation for the conflict. However, this kind of theatrical response, which engenders false and premature integration, may end up overlooking the main theme of the conflictual story. By separating the various voices, members are experimenting with the possibility of immersing themselves in and exploring a single voice, while allowing other members to represent the other voices. They are thus learning how to clarify the different voices, while the dramatic structure facilitates integration in a way that neither regulates nor diminishes any of the voices. This theatrical form is an invitation to fully integrate the different voices, as they arise from the paranoid-schizoid position, rather than attempt a partial and forced integration, which leaves many psychic parts weakened and beyond the scope of one's emotional experience. The integration achieved through this theatrical pattern contains the full emotional complexity of the conflict, rather than diluting it.

In many cases, the members portraying the opposing voices find it difficult to maintain the split for a long enough period of time and tend to rush to the dialogue much too soon. Nevertheless, this capacity to wait emphasizes that each side needs to clarify its place and its importance. The transition to dialogue can only emerge at a later stage. It is important to understand that, even during the stages of differentiation and clarification, integration is taking place by the very fact that the different voices are expressed together in the playing space, within a linking aesthetic structure. Only in this manner and toward the end of the theatrical response can the dialogue between the two voices potentially lead to the connection of two whole sides. Importantly, it is possible for the two sides to communicate without having to reach a premature solution or compromise. In many cases, change and growth are embedded in the very capacity to create such communication between the two sides. Moreover, the therapeutic effect is simultaneously present for both the playing members and the teller, because the possibility of exclusively inhabiting and maintaining a single position is a valuable psychic capacity. Often, this is a chance for members to explore voices that they avoid or tend to diminish and dissolve (such as voices that are aggressive, dismissive, dependent, etc.).

Consider the following vignette:

Teller: I'm going back to work after a year on sabbatical. On the one hand, I want to try new things, make some dreams come true, see what's exactly right for me. On the other hand, I want to go back to what is safe and familiar. Another dilemma is about the scope at which one should resume one's old job after a sabbatical.

Voice a (representing one side of the conflict): God save me from having to sell myself. There's no way I'm going down that road, start looking for scraps here and there, looking for people, heading out into the unknown. It's better to stay on the safe side.

Voice B (representing the other side of the conflict): I want to soar, to grow. I can see myself getting a master's degree, moving around, dreaming, doing, this is my chance, this time, I'm the one who's going to win, not my fears.

Teller's response: That's the story. They reflected my confusion by having both desire and fear together. Also, the body language of the two voices – the ease of the voice that stayed versus the unease of the worried voice. Right now, my decision is to stay conflicted. To understand. To stay undecided. I also think that I know the anxious side very well and, growing up, it was always made up to be important and wise. As if being a wise and responsible person means being an anxious person. I'm less familiar with the calmer side. I always think of it as some irresponsible "stoner." Now, I think that it, too, deserves to live. I have to say that this is making me nervous. I can really feel it in my body – that something bad might happen if I let my calmer side be more dominant, as if anxiety is my way of preventing catastrophe.

One behind the other

This pattern highlights and heightens the emotional force of the conflict. Unlike the "back to back" pattern, in which both voices are granted an equal amount of time to express themselves in a pure and uninterrupted way, this pattern features one voice being given front-center stage to share its position with the spectators and try to explain it. This position often coincides with the more socially accepted norm. Behind it, the more silenced voice – which usually represents instinctual motivations – is hiding. The frontal-social voice is hiding these silenced-instinctual parts, afraid that they might be revealed. For it, this other voice is a destructive presence that threatens everything the social persona has achieved through all its hard work. The frontal-social voice thus tries to keep the rear-instinctual voice from expressing itself, while the latter tries to find a way to break through into the playing space and reveal itself. This clash of opposing views creates a veritable struggle between two sides. This form serves as a therapeutic intervention in cases where the intensity of the conflict is denied and dismissed.

In this pattern, one playing member faces the spectators, while another member hides behind them. The member on the front represents the social side (a kind of super-ego) of the conflict. The member who is hiding represents the instinctual side of the conflict. The presentable side is trying to offer the spectators a learned lecture on the subject at hand, while the instinctual side is physically and verbally interrupting them with their instinctual expressions.

Consider the following vignette:

Teller: I've been working at the same job for 20 years, I don't enjoy it anymore and I feel suffocated. I sometimes think about leaving. I hardly ever share these thoughts with anyone else. You don't just get up and leave a safe and steady job, and besides, I've got a family and a responsibility.

Presentable voice (standing at the front of the playing space): I'm all set; I have a family, kids, a well-paying job, stability and a steady routine.

Instinctual voice (trying to break through): I have dreams (he goes on to express specific fantasies that the teller has shared in previous stories).

Presentable voice (quickly pushing the instinctual voice back): I've been at the office for 20 years, I have status, and I'm well respected. I only take on the projects that I want to do.

Instinctual voice (breaking through): I'm suffocating, I'm dying, I need air, and something has to change.

Presentable voice (blocking): Family comes first.

Instinctual voice (breaking through): I come first.

Presentable voice (blocking): Hush... you're going to get me fired, you egomaniac.

Teller's response: It was powerful suddenly watching that voice at the front of the stage desperately trying to keep the voice in the back from speaking. I thought about my own experience, and I often do feel suffocated, and I have all this anger that I can't understand. I don't know if I'm going to quit my job or not, but I realized how much I've been keeping myself from expressing this side, not communicating it to the people who are close to me, like my family, because I'm assuming they're going to be against it. And suddenly, after watching this, I'm not at all sure that keeping quiet is doing me any good... I was devastated by that part where he said "egomaniac." In my family, that was the worst insult for someone, being considered an egomaniac.

Cross

This conflict-presentation pattern emphasizes the element of potential integration and the co-existence of the two sides of the conflict. Unlike the other two patterns, in which the voices are heard separately or in mid-conflict, this pattern has both sides existing side by side and shifting the audience's attention between them. At some point, the two sides meet and engage in an exchange of ideas. This state often leads the teller to the realization that the two sides can be connected as two points on a single spectrum.

The two playing members decide which side of the conflict each of them is going to play. They both face the spectators, with one member standing on the right side of the playing space and the other on the left. The playing members are instructed to imagine that there is a kind of joining axis stretched out between them – and they slowly walk along this axis toward its center. At this point, they are constantly looking out at the spectators rather than at each other. Each player in turn delivers a single line, which presents their side of the conflict, and takes one step sideways toward the midpoint of the axis. In this manner, the two playing members are walking toward one another. When they reach the midpoint, they encounter each other. It is only at this stage that they first make eye contact. They dwell on this moment for several seconds, during which they rotate around an imaginary pivot and switch both their position on stage and their chosen side of the conflict. The playing members take turns continuing their motion along the imaginary axis, now moving away from each other, as each of them expresses the side previously expressed by their counterpart. They keep moving until each of them stops at the opposite end of the playing space. Because one of the drawbacks of this form is the tendency of playing members to limit their avenues of expression to the strictly verbal, it is important to emphasize the considerable significance that physical expression can have in this form.

Consider the following vignette:

Teller: I wanted to tell you about this dilemma I'm in. I'm at home with my kids and I love being with them. It's also something that's very important to me. On the other hand, I'm really thinking about going back to the job market to develop myself professionally and, what can you do, we need the money.

Voice A: Children are everything. The first years are crucial, they determine how they're going to turn out, what kind of people they'll be, and I just have to be there for them.

Voice B: I gave and I gave and now it's time to get back to myself. I'm very good at my job and I love it, too.

Voice A: I know but this is what is right for me, I can feel it deep down inside, how could I be away from them? How would they manage without me? They will to be terribly sad and so would I.

Voice B: I am sick and tired of this domestic routine. Honestly, it really isn't for me. I don't understand how other women do this; I need to get back to work as soon as possible, to get some sanity back.

The two voices meet and make eye contact. They revolve around their pivot and switch places. From this point on, the member who represented the first voice takes it upon himself to express the opposite viewpoint and vice versa.

Teller's response: This gave me a fresh perspective. Because, up until now, I felt that I had to make a choice, not leaving the house meant that my children would pay a dear price and that, if I wanted to focus on my kids, I would have to give up the things that are important to me. Now, I'm reminded of choices that my parents had made. Now, I understand that both these needs are a part of me and that I need to address both. I might even be able to be more at ease about spending time with my children. Otherwise, I would feel that I'm doing that at my own expense.

In conclusion, this chapter focused on the ability to observe opposing, ambivalent, sometimes paradoxical parts of human experience. The capacity to contain opposing aspects of the story within a single playing space results in an integrative experience of the self that contains the sum of one's qualities, attributes, roles and tendencies. The following chapter will discuss the potential for expanding one's range of looking at the story through the other.

Chapter 5

Expansion of the self through the other

Ronen Kowalsky, Nir Raz, Shoshi Keisari

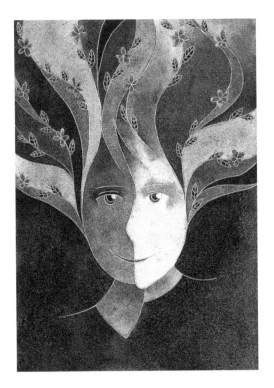

Figure 5.1

This chapter focuses on the group and the interpersonal process created in Psychotherapeutic Playback Theater. The group members both offer up personal stories to which others will respond theatrically and enact the personal stories of others. The theatrical response, which presents the personal experience portrayed by the story, creates a deep, emotional, immediate and

DOI: 10.4324/9781003167822-6

tangible encounter between self and other. This unique encounter establishes a transitional space, which unravels the self/other dichotomy. This is the foundation of the therapeutic process of Psychotherapeutic Playback Theater: *self-expansion through the other.*

Jonathan Fox, Jo Salas and the original Playback Theater group sought to create a meaningful form of social theater, which would bring about a true encounter between individuals and their stories. The force driving this encounter is the desire to expand one's personal story by letting it pass through the other via a theatrical response, which both mirrors and reinterprets the story's narrative. This is the origin of the name "playback," which expresses the tender way in which the story is passed from the teller to the stage and back again (Lubrani-Rolnik, 2009).

In this book, Psychotherapeutic Playback Theater is presented as a type of group therapy; as such, it is based on a form of thinking that is essentially group-oriented and intersubjective. Biran (2015a) perceives group therapy as taking place in the middle of the continuum between individual therapy and life itself. This is because, in individual therapy, the therapist "lends" herself to understanding the patient's subjectivity (Bion, 1970), becoming a sort of "transitional object," located between the patient's internal world and their projections onto reality and the otherness of the therapist (Winnicott, 1971). In group therapy, however, the patient encounters various perspectives and life experiences that differ from her own and that are, therefore, more likely to result in conflictual or confrontational interactions than in individual therapy. In group therapy, transitional space exists between all group members and between them and the conductor. Therefore, as Biran (2015a) suggests, individual therapy takes place in a more protected space than group therapy.

However, because Psychotherapeutic Playback Theater takes place within the context of a theatrical endeavor, which orients interpersonal space and interactions toward empathy and mutual understanding, it may be characterized as a type of group therapy whose level of safety lies between those of group therapy and individual therapy. Within the theatrical response, the playing member becomes, to a certain extent, a transitional object for the member telling the story, partially affirming Bion's (1970) injunction that the therapist should serve as an emotional "container" for the patient. At the same time, the story itself becomes a sort of transitional object for the playing member, who "borrows" the teller's story and uses it to make her own psychic discoveries.

Alongside its existence within a group therapy framework, a large part of the process of Psychotherapeutic Playback Theater takes place through the narratives introduced by group members. This creates a duality by which, while the personal story stimulates a group process, this process remains essentially committed to serving the individual teller. This commitment is crucial to the overall process and even ethically significant, considering the teller's vulnerable situation. In this sense, Psychotherapeutic Playback Theater calls for the integration of personal and group narratives, an aim which is far from obvious, given the constant tension between each member's belonging needs and individuation needs. The processing of this tension is a precondition for both intimacy (as full as possible self-expression in an interpersonal situation) and internalization (incorporating something originally experienced as "not me" into one's self).

Group members are constantly expressing a compelling need to both belong to the group and express their true self as fully as possible. These needs are often experienced as a conflict – a person may feel required to refrain from expressing certain parts of themselves in order to be accepted by the group. Alternately, they might feel the need to forego their sense of belonging to the group in order to express themselves more fully. The settling of this conflict is of the utmost importance; seeing as failure to do so diminishes one's capacity for both intimacy and internalization, which are essential to mental health, growth and the development of satisfying relationships with others. The basic feature of Psychotherapeutic Playback Theater – the development of the self by working with the psychic material of others – is precisely designed to help process this conflict.

Mirroring and the exchange of psychic material

In the Psychotherapeutic Playback Theater process, the development of the individual through the other group members is facilitated by the simultaneous presence of two main aspects: "playing the other" and "allowing the other to play me" (Kowalsky et al., 2019). Both these aspects express two of the main functions of group therapy, according to Foulkes (1964, 1990): mirror reaction within the group context and the exchange of psychological material.

These two aspects are demonstrated through a post-traumatic story shared in a Psychotherapeutic Playback group for holocaust survivors. One should note that, when dealing with stories that involve post-trauma, the reconstruction of the narrative, especially in terms of shifting it from a context of guilt toward a narrative of coping, is very important. While such reconstruction draws, in most cases, on the material of the teller's narrative, in this instance group members created a new narrative as a counterpoint to the teller's original story. We have chosen to present this particular vignette because it highlights the group's engagement in narrative intervention.

The story was shared by Isaac, a 75-year-old man, after having survived the holocaust as a child, immigrating to Israel, building a family and even heading various Zionist state-building projects. Nevertheless, he said that he found it very difficult to enjoy and relish his achievements and even revealed that he has never been able to sleep the whole night through. In one of the sessions, he spoke of the reason for these difficulties: when he was ten, during one of the Nazi raids, he tried to escape. He ran and hid in an attic. The Nazi soldiers came up to the attic and started looking for him. They came closer and closer to where he was hiding and, mere seconds before they would have found him, they pulled a screaming little girl from a different hiding place and shot her to death. In his mind, it was the girl's death that saved him. Ever since, whenever he starts feeling joy or pleasure, that little girl's screams begin to echo in his mind.

The group, whose other members also survived the holocaust as children, began the theatrical response with one member entering the playing space and, terrified, walking along its circumference looking for a place to hide. At some point, he grabs a dark piece of cloth, sits down in a chair, covers himself with the cloth and, shaking all over, whispers: "they're coming. They're coming. I was told to hide. I have to hide real well so that they don't catch me. I wish I could turn invisible. I want to disappear, so that they don't find me." At this point, another member enters the back of the playing space, she looks left and right in fear and then sits down and covers herself with a cloth as well. Then, two more members enter the playing space, their movements crude and heavy, and start looking by overturning chairs and throwing cloths around. They keep advancing toward where the girl is hiding but, at the last moment, change direction and move toward where "Isaac" was hiding. They remove the cloth from him. He tries to run but they grab him, hold him by the shoulders and lead him out of the playing space. Once outside, one of the two members who plays the Nazi soldiers bangs his hand on a table to simulate a gunshot. Then, the member who plays the little girl comes out of hiding, looks left and right and sneaks out of the playing space. At that point, a second gunshot is heard.

The playing members created a narrative in which the Nazi soldiers first find Isaac and shoot him and then shoot the girl as well. After the theatrical response, Isaac found it difficult to speak and it was clear that this new perspective he was presented with had rendered him speechless. The theatrical response stressed the fact that Isaac's survival had nothing to do with the girl's death and that his life and hers were not intertwined. This new scenario clearly showed that finding Isaac did not keep the Nazi soldiers from finding and killing the girl.

In some cases, the teller finds it hard to express their feelings after the theatrical response is over and it is up to the group to help find the words for these feelings through the sharing circle. Here, the other members shared a lot of feelings and stories about the theme of "survivor's guilt" – their guilt for having survived while others were left behind. One member talked about leaving a little girl behind. Another member talked about her father, to whom she was very close, and her difficulty in accepting the fact the she survived the war while he did not.

The following week, at the group's next session, Isaac shared that, for the first time in his life, he was able to sleep through the night. Later on, he reported that his ability to enjoy interacting with his wife, children and grandchildren has significantly improved. He mentioned the group's restructuring of his narrative as a crucial milestone in this process. The theme of "survivor's guilt" stayed with the group as a prominent motif over the next sessions.

The group's *mirror reaction* enables the individual to perceive himself, or parts of himself, mirrored back through group interactions. Through one's influence on others, one may come to know oneself better (Foulkes, 1964). In this manner, the theatrical response concretizes the act of mirroring by playing various aspects of their self back to the individual and allowing them to observe a picture of themselves as perceived by others. Foulkes (Foulkes & Antony, 1965) called this aspect of the group *the hall of mirrors*.

In the theatrical improvisation responding to Isaac's story, the mirror reaction is manifest in the presentation of narrative elements from the story, such as searching for a place to hide, running, tensely looking back, hiding, the soldiers' appearance and the shift in mood from fear and tension to terror. A highly significant part of the mirror reaction is the emotional change that the characters on stage underwent, along with the audience. The unfolding sense of terror was presented very vividly, evoking a deep sense of identification in the group members. The mirror reaction component provided the teller with a sense of recognition and an emotional connection with the playing members. The mirror reaction continued to reverberate throughout the group process created by the theatrical response, informing the sharing circle as well as the following sessions. In this instance, one could see how the theme of "survivor's guilt" became the center of the group's "hall of mirrors" by receiving many diverse mirror reactions from group members.

The *exchange of psychological material* is described as the possibility of sharing and transmitting material, much like the way a group of children plays together – one gives the other something from her inner world and the other gives her something back in exchange. Unlike the mirror reaction, which expresses and stresses the similarities between self and other, the group exchange of materials emphasizes the differences and gaps between self and other, highlighting these as an opportunity for self-development (Zinkin, 1993). The theatrical response expresses this therapeutic function by inherently taking place in the context of a creative encounter with the other. The materials of the story are processed in the minds of the playing members, whose inner world resonates that world suggested by the teller's words. The theatrical response is a collaborative creation which is born from this encounter.

The theatrical response embodies both the mirror reaction and the exchange of psychological contents (Foulkes, 1964, 1990). The personal story is introduced into the group, coming in contact with others and creating a collective, shared group experience. Through the theatrical response, which mirrors the story, its materials resonate in the minds of the other members.

In this regard, the theatrical response expresses the *mirror reaction*: mirroring different parts of the story and potentially echoing different meanings, amplifying emotional elements and offering validation and imparting a sense of value to the story and its themes. This creates a sense of universality in the group and the resulting notion that the personal story is part of the broader fabric of humanity provides one of the most important types of recognition in group therapy (Yalom & Leszcz, 1995). The group's mirror reaction creates a myriad of mirrors, in which each member reflects others and is reflected in their eyes. This strengthens the sense of belonging and intimacy, in the sense that each member both is seen by the group and contributes to its capacity to see others.

At the same time, the theatrical response expresses the *exchange of psychological material*, emphasizing differences between members and the growth-promoting potential of such differences (Zinkin, 1993). The other encounters the story, uses it to enter a playful space and offers different points of view. Through this process, the story takes on new meanings and dimensions, allowing fresh and varied perspectives to come to light in a way that enhances development for the entire group (Sajnani & Johnson, 2011). The story can be expanded because of the other's difference and the manner in which members exchange psychic materials in a creative-dramatic process, which unfolds in the group playground – the playing space. Thus, the theatrical response expresses commonalities and similarities between group members alongside its emphasis on exchange processes, which stress differences between members and the potential development these differences entail.

In the theatrical response to Isaac's story, the exchange of psychic material is manifest in the ability of the group members, themselves holocaust survivors who are thus deeply acquainted with "survivor's guilt," to offer at a later stage of the improvisation an alternative narrative, one that Isaac could not have created by himself. Isaac was carrying an immense sense of paralyzing guilt because he was holding on to a narrative by which he was saved because the Nazi soldiers caught the girl and spared him as a result. In fact, no one knows what might have happened otherwise. The choice the members made to present a different version of reality, in which his being caught by the Nazis before the girl had no effect on her survival whatsoever and she ended up being murdered either way, alleviated his feelings of guilt significantly.

The ability to simultaneously contain both similarities and differences between group members acts as a catalyst for group processes. While this promotes a sense of belonging, connection and involvement among group members, it also encourages reflective observation, which promotes their development. The mirroring of similarities offers an experience of recognition and validation and the normalization and universalization of personal experience. Universality and the sense of belonging are two of the main curative factors in group therapy (Yalom & Leszcz, 1995). Meanwhile, the validation of differences between members, in a way that emphasizes discrepancies between the respective experiences of the playing members and the teller, encourages confrontation processes, offering new insights and perspectives on one's personal experience. The constructive processing of this discrepancy is conducive to self-expansion, as it confronts one with unconscious and denied parts of one's self. In turn, this further expands one's self-awareness and the ability to internalize. These processes encourage growth and development for the teller, the other group members and the group as a whole (Schlapobersky, 2016).

Shifting between personal narratives and group narrative

One of the main ways in which the conductor can support the mutual nourishment of individual and group as well as resolve the conflict between belonging and individuation needs is by directing the movement between the individual's narrative and the group's narrative. This movement is created when personal narratives are processed and gradually interwoven into a group narrative (Kowalsky et al., 2019). The conductor can facilitate this process by incrementally reducing the relative time and space each story, with its unique language and characters, is given so that eventually, a group language can emerge and the different stories can slowly be woven into a shared tapestry. To this end, the theatrical response can be used to present more group narratives rather than individual narratives, highlighting the group process and space. For example, a member can share a story that deals with the experience of being seen (or not) by the group or a situation that involved conflict and tension with other group members. We recommended submitting these experiences to the creative theatrical process and processing them like any other experience or story introduced into the group space. It should be stressed that the shift from the personal voice to the group voice is not the end goal of the process and that it is important for the group to move back and forth between focusing on the individual voices of the members and reinforcing the group space. This is the only way to recognize, legitimize and address both the belonging needs and the self-definition and individuation needs of the members.

One of the most meaningful instruments the conductor in Psychotherapeutic Playback Theater has at their disposal when seeking to weave personal narratives and voices into a tapestry of group narrative is the act of *threading* (or finding the *red thread*). Drawing on the assorted materials introduced by group members, the conductor looks for a suitable theme or element that could tie this associative flow of material together and lend meaning to it. The process of threading is designed to create a container capable of holding the various contents in a way that offers unifying meaning, enhances group cohesion and increases the sense of mutual relevance among members. Threading is often performed after the *check-in round* (see below) and as the conclusion of the entire session. These moments in the session are specifically chosen as opportunities to increase the members' sense of group cohesion and mutual relevance, prior to moments of transition which undermine cohesion, such as the transition from going around the circle and hearing everyone's input to focusing on a single member's personal story or the transition from being in the session to the unraveling of the group as each member goes their separate way, back to their personal life, until the next session. The conductor is free to add additional points of threading throughout the session, in accordance with group needs. The act of threading the red thread is, in essence, a form of structuring and a way of working with the group container (for a more in-depth discussion, see the chapter on levels of structuring in Psychotherapeutic Playback Theater).

For example, during the sharing circle that followed Isaac's story and the theatrical improvisation responding to it, another member offered the metaphor of "life taxes": "I feel as if I have to pay a tax to those I left behind for every breath I take – I have to think about them and bring them back to life that way." Once the sharing circle was over and before returning to the teller, the conductor chose this metaphor of "life taxes" as the "red thread" that connects the different stories shared by the various group members:

I feel that this image of "life taxes" – there's a whole lot to it. This feeling that our life cannot be taken for granted but also that we have to pay for it by feeling guilty. As if it has been bought with suffering. And there is new notion here that maybe we can untie the knot that is binding the fact that we are alive to suffering and guilt; maybe we've already paid our dues and we can find a way just to live.

After the sharing circle and the above threading, the conductor turned to Isaac, who said:

I'm thinking of this phrase, "in their death, they commanded us to live."[1] Somehow, I'm managing to breathe differently with it right now.

The split between self and other – fact of life and illusion

The theatrical aspect of Psychotherapeutic Playback Theater creates a direct encounter between self and other, offering a paradoxical way of dealing with this fundamental and primordial split in human experience. This split is manifest throughout all stages of development, through fundamental questions regarding self-definition and defining the other; intimacy and alienation; abandonment and invasiveness; separateness and merger. To a certain extent, Psychotherapeutic Playback Theater challenges this self/other split in its attempt to bring down barriers and encourage psychological growth.

Bion (1970) defined psychic growth as the ability to learn from one's experience, to discover and understand something new. Knowledge that is grounded in the past can allow one to understand certain things about oneself, but not to grow or learn anything new. Real growth takes place through a dialogue with the other, which provides a novel perspective. Bion uses the term *vertex* (angle, point of view) to describe this and claims that the ability to attain psychological growth depends on an encounter that allows one to move between different points of view.

In Psychotherapeutic Playback Theater, having other people encounter and interact with one's personal story creates many new perspectives on one's experience. The playing member's encounter with the story creates a deep, experiential space of meeting with the teller. According to Bion, to create a true encounter with an experience, one must abandon one's pre-existing knowledge, past, memory and desire for satisfaction (of any need whatsoever, such as alleviating a symptom or replacing not-knowing with knowing), thus also abandoning the future. Bion defined this experience as "becoming O" (Biran, 2015 b), a state of utter at-one-ment with experience. Setting aside the past and the future enables clarity of mind and full connection to the "here and now," i.e., the truth. One gains access to an empty or "unsaturated" state, which facilitates investigation, observation and connection to the teller's experience. These moments, according to Bion, are a genuine opportunity for psychological growth and learning.

The Psychotherapeutic Playback Theater process involves precisely such an encounter, which encourages the individual to develop an emotional and experiential connection with the experience of the other. This is an invitation to enter a space that allows observation through dynamic movement between different vertices. One can move between closer points of view, which strive to accurately mirror the teller's conscious experience of their story, as well as between more distanced points of view, where playing members are more at liberty, offering more associative input. Most theatrical responses open with a perspective (vertex) that is relatively close to the teller's conscious emotional experience and eventually broaden their scope to include associations evoked by the personal story.

This embodies the essential idea that the story of the other offers an expansion of the story of the self. The individual's story resonates in the mind of the others, who respond to it from different points of view, both closer to and more distant from that of the teller. The opportunity to offer associations in response to the story expands it in a way that promotes the therapeutic process for both the teller and the playing members as the process of encountering a personal story encompasses the entire group. Although playing members are there to serve the teller, both in principle and in praxis, they cannot present and mirror the material of the story without first processing it through their own self-experience. This, in fact, leads to a developmental paradox: on the one hand, this is an immense developmental challenge, requiring the playing member to encounter both the contents of the story and their own inner world with empathic attention; they are then asked to use their own stories to resonate the story of the other, while translating both into the language of theater; finally, all this takes place through creative, playful processes which are inherently regressive.

This paradoxical situation makes Psychotherapeutic Playback Theater a unique form of therapy when it comes to working with projective identification. Ogden (1979) claims that the most meaningful level of therapy involves the therapist's ability to experience, contain and resonate the emotional material which is intolerable for the patient and thus distanced from their conscious experience. The therapist can thereby offer the patient a new opportunity to re-internalize these experiences and cope with them. In Psychotherapeutic Playback Theater, such development-promoting processes often occur within the playing space, through the working through and resonance of primary and unprocessed psychic material, as it is communicated by the teller to the conductor and the other members.

"The emotional experience is forced upon me, and I must experience it in a way that I cannot learn from and which I cannot remember," this is how Bion (1992) describes the process in which the patient "pours" unintelligible psychic material into the therapist. The role of the therapist – and thus also of the conductor and the performing members – is to make the unthinkable thinkable through an associative process Bion calls *reverie*.

Members are constantly transmitting nonverbal contents and unexplained emotions and feelings to one another. The conductor and the members feel each other absorbing each other's states of mind and being to varying extents. Because this mutual experiencing gives rise to feelings that are indicative of the other's experience, playing members may encounter diverse emotional contents such as being stuck and uncreative, unexplained sadness or anxiety. These feelings may be an echo of the unconscious psychic material of others, as expressed through the stories and introduced into the interpersonal interactions of the group. Playing members can draw on a variety of creative and artistic tools to express these experiences in the playing space, presenting such feelings directly or metaphorically, through verbal, visual or movement-based means. They may also quote existing texts and sing or play songs and melodies in a way that is associatively related to the experience, making it more explicitly and openly accessible.

The struggle between belonging and uniqueness

Throughout the group process, members experience an internal struggle between their desire to belong to the group and their need to maintain their individual uniqueness within the group. This struggle manifests itself as a conflict: belonging to the group involves the risk of losing one's individuality; maintaining one's individuality may require giving up one's sense of belonging. The therapeutic process strives to resolve this split and create an integrated experience in which the individual is not required to give up her identity in order to feel that she belongs.

In his play, *No Exit*, Jean-Paul Sartre (1949) presents the main tenets of his theory about the relationship between the individual and society. In the play, three characters await judgment in a room which is, in fact, hell. While they wait, the emerging dialogue shows their alienation from each other, which is so extreme it becomes insufferable. This is when the play's famous quote – "Hell is other people" – is delivered. According to Sartre, every relationship limits the individual's free, authentic self-expression, due to the discrepancies and misunderstandings inherent in all interpersonal communication. According to Sartre, the other's Otherness is the hell of the self. This description outlines a common fundamental difficulty: the threat the other presents to the authentic self leads to a difficulty in internalization, limits one's capacity for empathy, compassion and even understanding of the other and eventually halts the self's psychic growth. In contrast to Sartre, Levinas (1987) builds his theory of self-other relations around his notion of "the face of Other." In his view, all development – psychological, ethical and cognitive – is only possible to the extent that one is exposed to "the face of the Other" and is capable of withstanding both the gap between self and other and the distress this gap creates. These capacities are based on one's ongoing striving to dismiss the illusion that the other is or can be reduced to being the same as the self. Finally, development becomes possible as growth and correction of the self through the Other (Levinas, 1987).

In Psychotherapeutic Playback Theater, group members shift back and forth between *playing the other* – and thus being given the opportunity to experience, explore and hone one's ability to observe reality from the other's point of view – and *letting the other play them* – which uses the other to expand one's perspective on oneself. Through this process, group members are constantly practicing active engagement in intersubjective space, empathizing with and understanding the other. They are also acknowledging the satisfaction, the difficulties and the wish for correction this process entails. The group process thus highlights the encounter between self and other, which includes both elements that create the experience of growth and development and elements that create the experience of the other as hell.

Our individual identity emerges through our encounter with others. We often have no control over the most crucial factors that shape our identity: from our name to the nature and extent of the love expressed toward us to reinforcements and evaluation in terms of grades, admission exams, etc. Such dependence on others leads to anxiety, which surfaces whenever we encounter another person. Potentially, every such encounter entails the possibility, both exciting and unsettling, that a new experience of our self and our environment will emerge. This anxiety arises ever more sharply in the group process, which involves encountering multiple others as well as the big Other of the group itself. Similarly, the potential for attaining a new or recreated self-experience is more potent in the group. Finally, because many significant life experiences – whether extreme or routine, positive and growth-promoting or difficult and even traumatic – happen in the context of groups (our family, our schoolmates, our neighborhood, various institutions, etc.), we bring to the group session all these accumulated group experiences and their inherent potential for good or bad (Friedman, 2017).

Because the group process generates anxiety and poses a threat to one's self-esteem, the aim is to create a space where members can grow and internalize novel interpretations and points of view, facilitating a process of learning and developing through others. The theatrical response in Psychotherapeutic Playback Theater creates dynamic movement between different points of view and opens up a space for diverse interpretations. Its playful, flexible and creative form allows members to engage in self-expression and feel that they belong to the group space, while giving and receiving multiple, diverse interpretations.

Suggested session outline

In this section, we will suggest a possible structure for a regular session of Psychotherapeutic Playback Theater. Please note that its various elements are adjustable according to the conductor's preferences and the group needs. A typical session usually comprises the following stages.

The first stage, the *check-in round*, is designed to gauge both the emotional state of each member and the themes that emerge in the group process. During the check-in round, the conductor may mention those members who were tellers the week before. While the check-in round may be purely verbal, in time one can gradually add brief theatrical responses to the material being shared. These responses may address something in particular or combine several different issues or themes, thus serving as a theatrical threading. The use of theatrical responses in the check-in round may be done in a circle, through a round of movements expressing how each member is feeling at the start of the session. In another variation, each member offers a verbal sentence describing how they are that day and the other members respond with a movement that captures the psychic material they presented. Theatrical responses can be used to thread the different themes brought up during the check-in round. Such use of theatrical responses for threading the check-in round was found to accelerate the creation of a group container and the development of shared, relevant meaning for group members. This is because these brief responses transpose emerging material onto a more metaphorical level, thus expanding the meaning of concrete material, linking it to additional materials and finding a more global meaning.

The second stage of the session, the *warm-up*, is designed to make the group feel connected, playful and creative, facilitate interpersonal communication and listening and bring up materials and themes that would serve as the platform for the ensuing group processes. If the group feels stagnant, it is advisable to change up the order and try to introduce a sense of more dynamic movement by warming up before checking in.

The third stage is the *playback ritual*, where the group process unfolds through clear, predefined roles: conductor, teller, playing members and observing members. The conductor invites group members to volunteer, either as players in the theatrical response or as the teller, who will share a personal story. In certain cases, if the process takes place on a lower level of structuring, members do not volunteer in advance to play. Instead, the teller chooses a single member to portray the teller's character, while the other group members become potential players or observers (see Chapter 7).

Next, the teller sits on the designated teller's chair and tells their story spontaneously. The conductor can stop them and ask questions, in order either to expand the story or to focus it, as necessary. Then, after the conductor has asked the teller to find a *title* for their story, an improvised theatrical response is presented, in accordance with the conductor's preference, along the spectrum between improvisation and structure (a more or less structured pattern, several preplanned responses or a completely open improvisation; see Chapter 7). At this stage, playing members are required to practice empathic listening and try to portray the role of teller or of significant figures in their life, in an attempt to deeply embody the teller's personal experience. Once the theatrical response is over, the teller can react to it, ask to correct it or change certain elements.

Next, the group engages in a *sharing circle*, in which members can respond to the entire process of the ritual. The sharing circle addresses the need for mirroring and universality (Ryvko, 2018). Group members share the stories, feelings, thoughts and emotions that came up while listening to the teller's story and while presenting or observing the theatrical response. Thus, all members become involved in the process and share its materials, reinforcing their feelings of belonging, universality and cohesion (Yalom & Leszcz, 1995). The sharing circle concludes by returning the focus to the teller, who shares what they felt and experienced throughout the process.

At this stage, the task of the conductor is to thread the various materials and themes, whether introduced by the story or in the sharing circle, and link these to parallel group processes. In this manner, the presenting of a story and a theatrical piece responding to it create an immediate encounter between self and other, which is then observed and explored within the therapeutic space. Threading these materials and relating them to the parallel processes, taking place between the individual teller and the group and between group members, is significant because it creates a group container for the various psychic materials emerging in the group and increases the members' feeling of mutual relevance. These two aspects are vital for facil-itating the group process as simultaneous group therapy for all members, rather than merely individual therapy for the teller that utilizes the group. The conductor can perform the threading verbally or draw on the group thinking of the improvised process by borrowing images from one story to inform another and turning members' attention to potentially shared mean-ing. In our view, such interventions serve as a kind of modeling, encourag-ing members to mix and match images from different stories and thus play an active role in the quest for shared meaning and mutual relevance.

While the process of Psychotherapeutic Playback Theater revolves around the personal story of a single member, the fact that playing members can choose to portray certain roles from that story (rather than only being as-signed their role by the teller) and are free to offer their own interpretation of the story – through the improvisation and the encounter with personal material – creates an interactive, interpersonal group space in which the theatrical response takes place. In this fantastic space for action, the per-sonal experience presented in the story of an individual member becomes a collective experience that actively engages all members. One member's story encounters the stories of others and so everyone takes part in the thera-peutic process. Working through the other accelerates the group process and creates direct connections between members. In this manner, the entire process – from the warm-up stage, through the introduction of the personal story and the creation of a theatrical response to the final stage of the shar-ing circle – serve as a space that promotes *mental growth* (Bion, 1970).

Key elements in the Psychotherapeutic Playback Theater group process

In this section, we will discuss the key elements of the psychotherapeutic group process: attentiveness, action, the theatrical expression of transfer-ence processes, working through the relationship in the playing space, ex-plicit use of the conductor's subjectivity and working with the individual member.

Attentiveness

One of the most important tools that members of a Psychotherapeutic Play-back Theater group are required to hone and apply is *attentiveness*. The kind of active listening that enables actual contact with experience (Bion, 1970) begins from the outside and moves inward, toward the self. It requires one to "loosen one's screws" in order to open up to the full extent of the experi-ence. According to Bion, full contact with an experience occurs through the relinquishment of one's pre-existing knowledge (memory) and goals (desire) and the ability to tolerate the presence of an empty void – long enough for it to become full independently of one's needs and expectations. The idea is to direct one's attentiveness both inward and outward, creating a paradoxical experience in which listening outward means listening to the self. This movement reveals that listening to the other and being fully oneself are not contradictory.

Psychotherapeutic Playback Theater sessions often begin with statements such as "you've stayed with me all week," indicating deep internalization processes, the creation of dialogue and the questioning of previously held beliefs. While this experience is, in itself, positive and growth-promoting, by enabling a deep connection between self and other and potentially blurring the distinction between the two, it can also evoke anxiety. The conductor must be aware of such anxieties, which may involve both the fear of *engulfment*, which stems from such intermingling and mutual influence, and the fear of *abandonment*, which stems from the establishment of meaningful and valued relationships. Therefore, this deep encounter with the other offers an important opportunity to cope with and work through these fundamental anxieties, which are the main obstacles to creating intimate relationships and internalization processes. This can be facilitated by legitimizing the simultaneous processes of growing more intimate and merged and maintaining one's separateness.

Action

The first step in any process of change is action: the search for movement within a static state. Bion (1984) posits mental action, transformation, as the goal of the therapeutic process. He distinguishes between *thinking*, which is a dynamic, changing and evolving process, and *thought*, which is a mere static image. A thought may be a sort of way station in the thinking process, but it becomes a psychological problem when it remains immutable and precludes the dynamic flow of thinking. Bion describes a process in which the therapist must use her interpretations to spur the patient into action, into movement, into shifting from static thought to dynamic thinking. A similar process unfolds in Psychotherapeutic Playback Theater. The theatrical dimension operates through dramatic actions, which represent and work through the psychic material of the teller and the playing members. The teller thus shifts from a relatively passive position to a position that witnesses the transition into movement and the submission of psychic material to theater as an Other that stresses action and drama.

The playing members encounter their own personal materials by coming in contact with a story that is not their own. The very act of submitting the story and its psychic material to a theatrical framework of action requires them to transform static situations into active actions. Action itself generates change by creating a living, tangible experience in the "here and now" of the group. This experience takes place within a safe group space, utilizes significant others, offers new mirrors for the self and augments the personal experience brought up by the story. This parallels Fox's (1999) wish to use Playback Theater to establish the kind of theater that will be a platform for social change and a beacon of hope, where audience members are not passive spectators but the very heart of the process, inspiring the theatrical work.

The theatrical expression of transference processes

Playing members often experience different feelings and emotions in response to the material brought up by the teller. These feelings may surface while the story is being told, after it and during the creative process in the playing space. We view these feelings as transferential processes related to the teller and the materials introduced by their story. For example, feelings of detachment, being stuck or ill at ease, the emergence of personal associations or sudden spontaneity while improvising the theatrical response are manifestations of the players' encounter with the contents of the story and may prove significant for both the teller and the playing members themselves. For this reason, we encourage using these experiences within the creative theatrical process.

In a session of a Psychotherapeutic Playback Theater group, Debbie, a 26-year-old woman, talked about feelings of rage she is experiencing toward her manager at work.

> She keeps dropping so much work on me and I never even get the sense that she's grateful for anything I do. The only emails I ever get from her are ones asking for corrections or commenting on my work. In general, it feels like I'm working in a vacuum.

Yotam, a player with remarkable improvisational skills, entered the playing space and played Debbie's character. He started running about, organizing the chairs that were strewn around the room either in piles or in rows. Another member climbed up on one of the tables and, with a cold and arrogant tone, started giving him contradictory orders and occasionally criticizing him for something or other. At some point, Yotam stopped and tried to say something but was rendered speechless. He grew pale and it became clear that he was having trouble staying in the playing space. After the improvisation was over, he apologized and said, "that sucked. I don't know what came over me. I had an idea and then I just got stuck. This never happens to me. I was really unable to play." In response, Debbie said:

> the part where you were stuck is exactly the part that really stayed with me. It suddenly threw me back to when my father would scold me when I was a child. I would just stand there, dumbfounded and hope that it would pass.

Then Yotam added:

> I'm learning something from this, too. I usually feel that I can only go
> on stage if I have a good idea and when people go in without an idea and
> get stuck, I silently get angry. I suddenly remembered my own father
> who, when I brought home a test from school, would ask: "why just an
> A? Where did the plus go?"

This vignette illustrates the expression of transference relations in the improvisational process and their relevance for both the teller and the playing
members. One can see how the symbolic expression of these transference
relations in the playing space often creates distancing which allows for a
more comprehensive exploration of these relations.

Working through relationships in the playing space

After listening to the story, group members portray its dramatic roles and
relationships in the playing space. To a great extent, group work in Psychotherapeutic Playback Theater is centered on relationships in the "here and
now" of the group. The relationships portrayed in the playing space parallel
those expressed in the individual's story and the theatrical response enables
the simultaneous processing of these corresponding relationships. This is
done through the capacity of theatrical images to create transitional space
for these relationships, allowing for movement, change and growth. The encounter with the other invites an interaction that is full of stimulating and
surprising moments, giving rise to feelings of pleasure, belonging, surrender
and anxiety. In this space, one can explore the relinquishment that is a precondition for relatedness as well as the mourning processes that accompany
it. The playing space thus often sees the emergence of relations that serve
as a corrective experience for one's early relations with one's family of origins. This correction is one of the most significant therapeutic factors in the
group process (Yalom & Leszcz, 1995).

In a Psychotherapeutic Playback Theater group, Nufar, a 30-year-old
woman who looks and feels younger than her age, is being consistently
typecast as the "little girl" – both in group interactions and in the roles
she is given when improvising. She often ends up playing young, childlike
and naïve characters, who need the guidance and support of more ma-
ture figures. She herself often points out the fact that she is the youngest
person in the group. In contrast, 65-year-old Batya assumes the role of
the group's "all-knowing tribal elder" – a worldly wise woman who could
offer advice about anything. In the theatrical responses, she is often given
maternal, guiding and instructing roles. She tends to get into conflicts
with the conductor and has a lot to say about the decisions he makes in
the group.

In one session, Daniel, a 42-year-old man, talked about feelings of help-lessness in his relationship with Yaron, his 17-year-old son:

> A few days ago he just snapped at me, out of the blue. I couldn't under-stand what happened. He told me I was a shitty father and that all my criticizing has made him insecure, that I never believed in him. Then I snapped back at him, saying that I'm giving him my whole life and that he only knows how to complain and that I don't know what to do with him anymore. Then he suddenly started crying and ran out the door. We looked for him everywhere, checked with his friends and it took a long time before we found him. I really regretted what I had said to him. I thought that he was going to do something crazy. And when we finally found him, I couldn't stop myself and I snapped at him again. I'm so ashamed of myself.

For the theatrical response, the group chose the short pattern of a "duet": Batya chose to play Daniel while Nufar chose to play Yaron and the two stood side by side, facing the audience. As Daniel, Batya began a mono-logue, explaining to the audience how Yaron was never able to stick with anything he did and how that worried him. At some point, Nufar as Yaron interrupted this monologue and started a monologue of his own that de-scribed feelings of failure in relation to his father – "he's never happy with anything I do." After about a minute, Batya interrupted Nufar and, as Dan-iel, shared how difficult the events of the story were for him: "I don't know what to do with him." Then, Nufar interrupted her and, as Yaron, started another monologue: "I can't take it anymore. I'm being treated like I'm worthless, I have to get out of this house." They continued with these mu-tually interrupting monologues until the improvised response was over. In the Duet pattern, the characters both talked directly to the audience, rather than to each other. After the response ended, Daniel said to the conductor: "that was very accurate – that rift between us. It's like we're each in a sepa-rate world." He then added: "I feel that I need something more, that it can't end this way. I need help to understand this better."

In response, the conductor suggested that Batya and Nufar continue the improvisation, this time with a "Cross" pattern. Just like the "Duet" pat-tern, the Cross features two characters delivering mutually interrupting monologues to the audience. However, they are gradually moving toward one another until they meet halfway, make eye contact, circle an imaginary axis and undergo a transformation so that each takes on the other's role. In the first part of the improvised response, Nufar and Batya, in their respec-tive roles as Yaron and Daniel, said more or less the same things they had in the Duet pattern. However, when they reached the point where they had to make eye contact and change roles, the two froze for a moment. It became clear that this switch was taking both of them out of their comfort zone and confronting them with their personal difficulties. Nufar now had to portray an authoritative parental figure, who is concerned for his son and whose efforts to push his son to greater achievements have backfired. Batya now found herself playing the role of a rebellious and insecure teenager, who is fighting for recognition and for the sense that he has his own voice.

After this part was over, Daniel said:

> this was really strange. It gave me plenty of things to think about. I suddenly remembered the way I was at Yaron's age – I only cared about getting away from home, everything my parents did got on my nerves. And how insecure I was. I never thought I'd end up in this situation with my own son.

During the sharing circle, Batya and Nufar talked about the great difficulties they experienced when it came time to switch roles. Nufar said:

> I had to look for it inside myself and I was certain that I didn't have it in me – someone who knows what they're saying, who has to take responsibility over another person, how hard and how serious that can be – and having been able to do all that is a really powerful experience.

Batya said:

> I thought about my daughters and about myself as well – how hard it is for me to be in this place of not knowing. That's why I always have to know more than everyone else. It's so exhausting sometimes. I don't want people to think that I'm stupid and this took me back to times when *I* really thought I was stupid.

This vignette shows how Nufar's and Batya's respective ranges of potential roles have expanded through their interaction in the playing space, in the context of their shared encounter with Daniel's story. The role-exchange part of the "Cross" pattern confronted them with a significant and emotionally charged role that they had been avoiding and gave them the opportunity to draw inspiration from one another in the process.

The emphasis on parallel relationships also means that the conductor can take the teller's story at face value and as indicative of interpersonal relationships in the group. For example, if a member shares a story whose central theme concerns her place at work and not feeling seen there, this theme can be seen to represent a group voice that expresses the unseen or unnoticed part of the group or of each of its members, a part that is looking for ways to be seen and heard.

The check-in round is important because its materials permeate the emerging personal stories and encourage members to construe these as collective

stories that belong to the group as a whole. The use of symbols in the theatrical responses in Psychotherapeutic Playback Theater also reinforces the
interconnectivity of stories and highlights the simultaneous presence of the
personal and the collective. The conductor must therefore be simultaneously
attuned to both the story and the group process, which unfolds alongside
it and is embodied by it. This broadens the discourse surrounding group
dynamics as well as the group dynamics themselves. Because members naturally tend to avoid talking about their interpersonal relationships in the
group – due to anxiety, embarrassment, the fear of offending or being of-
fended, etc. – the conductor plays a crucial role in navigating the transition
between the personal and collective levels. As mentioned, the conductor's
aim is to harness the interpersonal dynamic in the group, both in the playing
space and outside of it, to promote relationships that offer a corrective experience for members' primary family relationships (Yalom & Leszcz, 1995).

Explicit use of the conductor's subjectivity

In some situations, the conductor may choose to openly utilize their own
subjectivity as an intervention, as part of the process of Psychotherapeutic
Playback Theater. This can be done by joining their personal voice to the
sharing circle or by taking part in an open theatrical improvisation. Such
direct participation must be done in moderation and with caution and must
take into account the group's specific situation and stage of development.
The conductor must make it very clear to the group that she is sharing her
own subjectivity in her role as the conductor, offering it as an intervention
and a sort of interpretation to the group. She must therefore be mindful
of how this intervention affects the group and make sure this is not done
impulsively. When choosing to take part in the theatrical response, the
conductor may do so in a number of ways: through verbal expression; by
amplifying a meaningful voice that is weak or absent; by introducing a unifying image that holds the different voices arising in the group; as an act of
threading performed within the theatrical response itself; or by introducing
an image from another story, in order to stress its connection to the present
story. It should be noted that, even when the conductor's intervention in the
improvised response is strictly interpretative, it still contains a prominent
component of self-disclosure.

In a Psychotherapeutic Playback Theater group, Shlomit, a 32-year-old
woman, talks about a recurring feature of her Friday-night dinners with her
parents and older brother. Every time the family sits down to dinner, the
conversation ends up being about Shlomit's frustrating difficulties in finding
a life partner. At that point in the evening, her brother starts telling dirty,
sexist jokes at her expense and her father joins in on the "fun," laughing
to himself. Then, her mother finds some excuse to leave the table, leaving
Shlomit to face her brother and father all by herself: "I wish I could just

disappear off the face of the earth. They're both so mean and nasty and I can't bring myself to talk back to them." The theatrical response began with two men members who entered the playing space and started telling a series of dirty, sexist jokes. It soon became evident that the two were relishing this opportunity to be on stage and say things that are considered unacceptable and provocative. The scene went on and on and no other member came in to add to it or change it. It felt like these two men were filling the playing space with their self-indulgence and even egging each other on to greater obscenities. Meanwhile, the teller could be seen shrinking in her seat and the entire group became paralyzed. At some point, the conductor entered the playing space and started saying, in a loud voice that soon grew to a shout: "this isn't my story! This isn't funny! You're both disgusting! Shut up already! You're unbearable!"

At that moment, the theatrical response was halted and there was a sense of awkwardness in the air. The teller said: "you really saved that for me. If it had just kept going that way, I would have ended up leaving the group. It was really unbearable. When you started yelling at them, I started breathing again." As for the two playing members, they expressed a great deal of anger at the conductor: "as we see it, you just broke the rules. It felt personal. It was you, as the conductor, coming on stage and shutting our mouths." The conductor then shared that, when he entered the playing space, he was shouting at the two men's characters both as the teller and as himself.

> It took me back those moments in high school, in the army, when people tell jokes that are not only dirty and sexist but also objectifying and belittling, and I always felt that I wanted to say something or just get up and leave – but I always ended up keeping my mouth shut and staying. I think that the most difficult thing for me was the way that both myself and the group stayed silent about what was happening here. I felt like I had to break this muteness.

During the sharing circle, one of the two playing members told the group how, as a child, he had joined his classmates in mocking a girl who was the class pariah. Another member talked about being disappointed in herself as a woman for needing a man to "save" her and speak on her behalf. Once the sharing circle was over, the teller said: "something really strange is happening here for me. As if something about these clear divisions into men and women is being a little undermined in my mind."

Just like any other group member, when the conductor enters the playing space, they speak through a character, while also speaking with their own voice. Just as one cannot view group members in the playing space as merely "playing a role," so the conductor is also exposing and expanding parts of themselves through their dramatic work. The conductor must be aware of this process and find ways to turn such self-disclosure into a part of the therapeutic process and an opportunity for further growth for the entire group.

Our experience in Psychotherapeutic Playback Theater has taught us that intersubjectivity is neither an approach nor a choice, but a clinical fact. Theatrical response takes place in a space that could only exist as an intersubjective encounter. The mindful movement of listening both inward and outward, performed by the conductor and the group members, reveals the intersubjective nature of this space. In fact, all of the conductor's interventions and considerations stem from their subjectivity; there is no other option. The question they are faced with concerns the extent to which they decide to reveal this process to the group. In order to answer this question, the conductor must try to determine whether the group has reached a sufficiently developed stage to be able to benefit from this expression of subjectivity or whether such subjective expression will be experienced as invasive and overburdening, thus preventing regression – which might have significant therapeutic ramifications.

Working with the individual

Relationships, by their very nature, involve anxiety about having to sacrifice one's uniqueness and individuality for the sake of belonging. In the Psychotherapeutic Playback Theater process, it is therefore important to emphasize each member's uniqueness as a separate individual alongside the process of expanding the self through the other. When a story is introduced into the group, it creates an important dialogue between the conductor and the teller that allows the teller to present their experience and give it their own personal mark. This is done, for example, by the conductor asking the teller to give the story a title, which motivates the teller to define what they see as the story's core. In certain cases, in order to allow the teller to maintain control of the story, they are given the opportunity to choose who will play their character and other characters in the theatrical response. Even after control of the story has been ceded to the playing members, who add new perspectives that expand the existing vertex (Bion, 1970), once the theatrical response is over, the conductor "returns" the story to the teller, asking them to respond to the resulting theatrical piece. The teller then shares what they have experienced while watching the response.

The tellers' experiences are varied and always serve as fertile ground for further exploration. In accordance with the teller's response and any new material they may share, the conductor may intervene in several ways: asking the teller to specify their needs and suggesting that the playing members perform another theatrical response to create a piece that is better adapted to these needs; asking the teller to change, adjust or add any material that was missing or share any new insights inspired by the theatrical response that they would like to see come to life in the playing space. Another possibility is to observe the process through the group discussion of the *sharing circle*, as an opportunity to process the story through the collective lens of the group and the individual lens of each individual member. As mentioned, in the sharing circle, members react to the story and the theatrical response and bring up any personal stories inspired by this process. When the teller hears experiences that resemble their own, this supports the transition from isolation to communality. The purpose of the sharing circle is to offer the teller an experience of universality. In many cases, members report feeling shame and anxiety about their story, which are considerably relieved during the theatrical response and especially during the sharing circle: "it is as if the story takes you out of the human race and Playback brings you back in."

In conclusion, the foundation of the therapeutic process of Psychotherapeutic Playback Theater is a deep and playful encounter with the psychic materials of others. This chapter described how this encounter facilitates the discovery of new aspects of the self. In addition, the chapter discussed the different stages throughout which this deep encounter is created as well as the inherent potential of each stage to promote new insights and discoveries. In the following chapter, we will discuss the area in which this encounter takes place and the different therapeutic qualities of the "playing space," the "stage" and their integration.

We will now present a warm-up exercise that expresses the notion of expanding the self through the other.

Shared dance

While playing upbeat music in the background, the conductor encourages members to begin moving about the room. After several minutes, the conductor asks members to form pairs, with one person leading the pair's movement and the other following and imitating – just like in a classic mirror exercise. The members of each pair spontaneously switch the roles of leader and follower, so that one is leading the movement and the other is mirroring them at all times. This creates a shared dance: synchronized movement that connects the two members. After they have practiced this for several minutes, the conductor can ask the different pairs to start joining up and make groups of four. In each of these groups of four, one person leads the movement, while the others mirror them. As before, the lead is spontaneously passed between them until each person has had their turn. Next, two groups of four will come together to form a group of eight and the exercise is repeated in the same manner. These groups of eight eventually join to encompass the entire group and the exercise is repeated, again, with one person leading the movement at any given time.

The principle of movement which involves the shifting roles of leader and follower, teller and responder is at the core of Psychotherapeutic Playback Theater. Simply by moving together around the room, the pairs have already begun the constant, ongoing exchange of roles, with one person leading a spontaneous-creative movement and another responding to the material they introduce. This exercise releases members from having to be responsible or to know how to do something. Some call this exercise "how to teach someone to dance, who doesn't know how?" The answer it offers is "through imitation." Responsibility and embarrassment are transferred to the other, enabling a state of playfulness in which everyone moves together. Imitation is thus a basic strategy designed to enable self-expansion through the other. Each member finds themselves dancing in ways they did not anticipate, by following the movements of the other. In addition, this experience involves mirroring, by allowing each member to experience themselves as they (their movements) are perceived by others. This mirroring creates an experience of being seen, recognized and valued. Throughout the exercise, the conductor must try to keep self-judgment and self-consciousness to a minimum, in order to cultivate the ability to create an uninhibited playing space and reduce awareness of the performative aspect of this activity.

Note

1 Translator's note: this phrase, a quote from a poem by Bialik, recurs often in Israeli discourse surrounding Holocaust memorial day and memorial day.

Chapter 6

From the playground to the stage

Ronen Kowalsky, Nir Raz, Shoshi Keisari

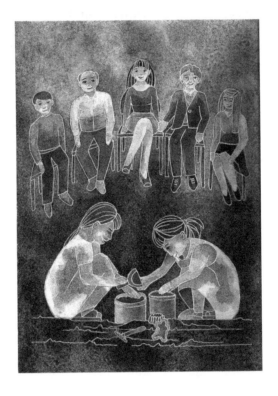

Figure 6.1

Psychotherapeutic Playback Theater seeks to create the primary and instinctual "playground" of childhood within the space of the "here and now." This playground is a spontaneous space, which facilitates the linking of fantasy and reality. This space, which Winnicott (1971) calls "transitional space," exists within the intermediary area between self and other, fantasy

DOI: 10.4324/9781003167822-7

and reality, and enables playfulness, spontaneity and creativity. Winnicott and the many other psychoanalytic authors who followed in his footsteps (Huizinga, 1949;Kulka, 2013; Lurie, 2013) have posited the capacity for play as a vital precondition for normal psychic development, for one's experience of aliveness and joy and for the ability to engage in creative interaction with others and oneself: "it is in playing and only in playing that the individual child or adult is able to be creative and to use the whole personality, and it is only in being creative that the individual discovers the self" (Winnicott, 1971, p. 54).

In its original form, Playback Theater is grounded in the principles and conventions of theater, which involve a clear distinction between the audience and the actors, who are watched as they perform on stage. While Psychotherapeutic Playback Theater takes place in a closed, ongoing group, the terms and experiences of "players," "audience" and "stage" are still relevant to it: the players and the audience comprise the group members, who are constantly changing roles. The stage is a certain space in the room which has been defined as the part of the therapeutic setting in which theatrical responses take place.

Various approaches in drama therapy have explored the beneficial potential of performing a piece of theater in front of an audience. The piece can be created over time or be improvised instantaneously (Pendzik et al., 2017). Being able to tell one's story to the group, to watch the theatrical image created in response to that story and to take part in creating this image allow members to experience a vital process which Kohut (1977, 1984) called *emergence*. This enables the tangible expression of parts of the self to others. The process of emergence exists for the teller, as they tell their story to the group, and it becomes even more potent through the theatrical response, which arises in response to this story. For the playing members, this process is manifest through their expression of their own creativity as well as the way their own psychic materials surface in front of the other members, through their response to the story.

The process of emergence can be likened to an actor standing on stage in the dark. They are unseen; they are in a place that, while safer and more protected from the threat of external observation and self-consciousness, is frustrating in terms of the desire to be seen. The very thing that keeps them safe also prevents them from being visible to others. Feeling unseen or invisible may sometimes lead to the feeling that one does not exist. In the process of emergence, a beam of light is cast on the player, making them feel simultaneously more present and more exposed. The capacity to be seen by a supportive and empathetic audience is an essential part of the development of the self (Kohut, 1977, 1984). Such a process is vital for the development and furtherance of healthy narcissism. Sajnani (2012) had stressed the importance of witnessing for both the witness and the witnessed, creating relational aesthetics, and by that enabling development and growth in the personal as in the social level.

First and foremost, however, standing in front of an audience often involves a high level of anxiety and a sense of being persecuted by the observing object, which may manifest as a heightened preoccupation with the quality of one's performance and the manner in which one is perceived by the observing object, i.e., the audience. Such critical self-observation often affects one's ability to draw on one's theatrical and creative capacities, which are so vital to psychotherapeutic processes (Winnicott, 1971), an ability which is prominently important and present in Psychotherapeutic Playback Theater. In many cases, group members in Psychotherapeutic Playback Theater are reluctant to join the theatrical response due to critical thoughts concerning its end result. These thoughts, which are often related to painful past experiences that involve feelings of shame or rejection, cause members to prefer to hide themselves, to remain in darkness and keep away from the spotlight. This blocks their ability to play and, along with it, the process of emergence, which is crucial for development.

In the group's very first session, during the opening circle, in which the conductor has asked members about why they chose to attend the group, Yoni, a 32-year-old man, shared that his first memory of public speaking was from third grade. The teacher had called him up to the blackboard. At that moment, he had felt very excited, "as if my heart was pounding so hard that I couldn't hear anything else." The teacher then asked him to write a few words on the board. Yoni felt 40 pairs of eyes piercing his back – "it was like needles being jabbed into my back." Ever since that incident, Yoni avoided any form of public speaking. For example, in his present workplace, he always found various excuses to keep from giving presentations before his colleagues and his bosses. Yoni says that he came to the group with a great deal of fear, on the one hand, and a strong desire to finally face this fear, on the other.

> I saw a Playback performance and, suddenly, I wanted to be up there on stage with them, so free and loose, improvising – but I immediately said to myself, "oh, you and your stupid ideas." And then I thought that I was sick and tired of this fear, that has been keeping me paralyzed my whole life, tired of living in its shadow. That's why I'm here.

Yoni's story illustrates the way a narcissistic injury has been playing a key role in shaping his life. Yoni eschewed and avoided the persecutory gaze of an imagined internal audience, while at the same time being drawn to the reparation manifest in a positive experience of emergence. Yoni's loaded ambivalence toward the stage demonstrates both the challenge and the therapeutic potential of creating a playful space alongside an experience of emergence and visibility.

This chapter discusses the various ways in which one can create playful and spontaneous experiences in a space that involves being visible to others – bringing the "playground" to the "stage," thus also turning the stage into a space of exploration and experimentation. In our view, the possibility for engaging in spontaneous and creative play even in a situation that entails a high degree of visibility is incredibly significant psychotherapeutically. Quite often, the split between the potential for authentic self-expression and the experience of emergence and visibility leads to a splitting of self-states. Thus, one on side of the split there are self-states that are experienced as false, because they are outwardly oriented and involve the wish to be seen and acknowledged; on the other side, there are self-states that are experienced as authentic, yet shameful and therefore hidden. The latter are often experienced as "the bitter truth," as authentic aspects that, had they been visible and made public, would lead to the person's rejection by others (Bromberg, 1993). Therefore, the ability to enable a space in which playfulness and creativity allow authentic self-states to emerge in a theatrical space of visibility is of the utmost therapeutic value. It allows various self-states to emerge and be acknowledged, validated and valued, while they are being presented on stage before a supportive audience.

In Psychotherapeutic Playback Theater, it is important to view the presence of the audience and the stage as two points on a single spectrum, which can be repositioned along this spectrum according to the group's needs (see Figure 6.2) (Kowalsky et al., 2019). At one end of the spectrum, there are forms of conducting that highlight the playing space as a *playground*, blurring the distinction between audience and stage. This happens, for example, when the large group is divided into small groups (containing three or four members). During such creative processes in small groups, each group picks which member will tell their story and which members will perform, switching roles after each story. Work in small groups also dedicates a distinct part of the playing space to the theatrical response – playing members play in front of one or two members who are watching them, thus creating a certain audience-stage distinction. However, the stage is less present when working in small groups: because there are fewer members, the playing space is smaller, its boundaries are less delineated and all members are actively and explicitly emotionally involved in the action. They all tell stories, experiment, act and share – changing roles relatively often. Accordingly, their dialogue is more explicit and their potential for experiencing freedom, playfulness and creativity – and even a certain degree of emergence – is very high. This kind of experience may reduce their level of persecutory self-observation or help them find better ways to handle such presence, facilitating a sense of capability and self-worth and eventually realizing the potential for performing in front of others. This leads to the gradual development of an experience that opens up a possibility for feeling emergence while accepting precisely those parts of the self that are hidden or silenced.

At the other end of the spectrum, we have forms of conducting that highlight the existence of the *stage* as a space that distinguishes between performers and spectators. These forms are more similar to the setup of Playback Theater shows. The teller shares their story while sitting in the audience with the other group members. Those members who have been assigned as playing members create a theatrical response in response to their story, in a space within the room that has been designated as a stage. Such forms potentially invite members to cope with a higher level of persecutory self-observation and to have a more significant experience of overcoming it as well as of visibility and emergence.

Psychotherapeutic Playback Theater sessions sometimes utilize the circle as a form. The circle is located somewhere in the middle of the abovementioned spectrum. It is a state in which playfulness moves around the circle, each time calling on a single member or several members to perform for the rest of circle. In this setup, all members are visible to all other members at the same time and the focus of the group's attention shifts between all of them. The circle setup can be changed according to the group's needs (e.g., performance can take place inside the circle or at its circumference; by a single member or several). The circle allows the conductor to make slight adaptations to the setting in order to heighten or diminish the presence of the distinct playing space: work inside the circle, for example, increases its distinct presence vis-à-vis the spectators, in contrast with work on the circumference of the circle, where the distinction between playing space and observation space is less pronounced; similarly, when several members work together in the circle, the sense of distinct presence is decreased, as compared to when a single member performs for everyone else (a more complete description of working in circles will be given below).

It is important to note that the possibility of performing in front of others should by no means be viewed as a given or taken for granted. Rather, one must gradually and carefully build up the group members' sense of capability and self-worth in preparation for such performance. An example of this can be seen in the work of a Psychotherapeutic Playback Theater group at a center for holocaust survivors. Leah, an 82-year-old woman, shared that, at the age of three, her parents, whom she barely knew, gave her away to the convent in which she hid during the war. She was given a strict upbringing by the nuns, who kept her Jewish identity hidden from her. She said that, once the war was over, when she found out that she was Jewish, she realized why they had treated her far more harshly than any of the other girls at the convent.

> I felt that that was some flaw in me, something that had to be taken out of me, and I never understood what it was. I felt that I had to excel in comparison to others in order to atone for some unknown sin.

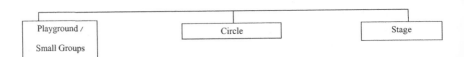

Figure 6.2 Levels of stage/audience presence.

Leah's need to excel was apparent in her adult life, as well. At the center, she repeatedly volunteered in various positions and took on much more responsibilities than others. In the group, she found it very difficult to improvise with her peers and it seemed like something was constantly holding her back on stage. She was overly critical of herself and others – "I don't understand what we're doing here. This isn't even theater. Someone tells a story and we do all kinds of things... I don't see the point." In addition, Leah gave off a general sense of being embarrassed in front of the other group members. Through her words, Leah was demonstrating how her space of visibility demanded that she should "perform" and excel, thus limiting her ability to play and enjoy an experience of aliveness, creativity and spontaneity.

The group's transition from working on stage to working in small groups led to a change in Leah's behavior. Working in small groups, in which each member plays the roles of actor, spectator or teller, made her more willing to experiment with the creative process, both as a teller and as an actor. This minimized her awareness of the presence of a stage and an audience, thus allowing Leah to surrender more fully to the playful and spontaneous experience of discovery – she started having unexplained little giggling spells and her work became more emotional and less controlled. She made more use of cloths, body and physicality and resorted to verbal expression less often. One could see Leah get carried away in the improvisational flow. Little by little, it became evident that working in the "playground" of the small groups diminished the presence of the internalized demanding audience in her psyche and enabled her to develop an increasingly free and creative playing space. In one of the sessions, Leah had a fit of long and rolling laughter; no one in the group had ever witnessed her laughing so hard. At the end of that session, during the final sharing circle, Leah said:

> I feel that this is the first time in my life that I have ever played. There is a lot of talk here about "playing..." "playing..." and I've always treated it with a little disdain. I think today I finally realized what it means.

Leah's case illustrates how important it is for the conductor to consider the aspect of playfulness in a member's process and the motion along the spectrum between the playground and the stage. Ignoring this aspect might mean abandoning group members to the mercy of their ferocious persecutory self-observation. This, in turn, can lead either to anxious avoidance of performance, to the extent that the member might leave or be excluded from the group, or to a brilliant and astounding dramatic display during the theatrical response. This display, however, conceals the cultivation of a well-functioning false self, while those parts of the self that tend to give rise to shame and anxiety remain silenced (Winnicott, 1965). The use of different levels of structuring, diverse theatrical forms and circle games are all milestones in the development of the group-play process on stage.

In his paper "Confusion of the Tongues between the Adults and the Child," Ferenczi (1933) argues that one of the mistakes made in psychoanalysis with adult patients is the assumption that one is indeed dealing with an adult patient, while two patients have, in fact, entered the room – the adult and the child hiding inside them. The adult may benefit from insights and self-reflection, while the inner child is mostly preoccupied with the actual, non-symbolic relationship between themselves and the therapist and the wish for a corrective experience to be achieved through the therapist's love for them. In Ferenczi's view, only if the inner child feels loved and safe can the adult truly benefit from the self-reflection and insights obtained in therapy. When the needs of the inner child go unnoticed and are left unaddressed, this leads to a "confusion of tongues," pseudo-therapy and another traumatization. In the present context, it is important to understand that the performance situation often touches on the traumatic experiences of that inner child, which reinforce regressive processes.

This is illustrated in the case of Ronit, a 42-year-old woman, whose mother gave her up to adoption when she was only a baby. As a child, she passed between various institutions and foster families and was only able to find a limited feeling of "being home" during her military service. She eventually started a family and now has two children; she is very devoted to her role as a mother and is even doing well at her job. In the group, during the sharing circles that followed the theatrical reflections – both of her own stories and the stories of others – she repeatedly complained about inattention and a lack of empathy – "I feel like the people here don't really care about each other and are just looking for a laugh." Some of the group members were empathetic toward Ronit and some even resonated their own sense of non-belonging and feeling alienated in the group – which was reflected on stage as a group theme. Nevertheless, Ronit's ongoing discontent gave rise to significant difficulty and even rage in the group. Ronit ended up feeling more and more alone and misunderstood. Even though the group made ample room for her feelings, after the sessions ended, she stayed behind to talk to the conductor, lengthily describing her feeling that both he and the group are not seeing her.

Ronit's relationship with the conductor began taking up more and more space – through phone calls and even individual sessions. In these conversations, she directed a lot of aggression toward the conductor – aggression which, until now, had been left uncontained by figures in her past who rejected her and could now be contained by the conductor. In one of these sessions, she even said, "I don't understand how, after a conversation like the one we just had, you're saying 'see you at the next session.'" In the group sessions, she talked about how her focus during the theatrical reflections is directed at the role of the conductor and how important his empathy is to her.

The notion that Ronit was expressing group material involving the experience of persecution on stage led the conductor to try and integrate more work in small groups during the sessions. One could see how working in small groups made it easier for Ronit, by limiting the scope of her projections and augmenting her ability to feel other people. Ronit herself mentioned that she felt more comfortable in the smaller groups and was more able "to get to know the people and get close to them." It was evident that she treated the members of her small group as individuals even back in the large group setting – addressing them by name, recalling personal things they shared that she could identify with or associating them with beneficent figures in her life. In one of the sessions, Ronit said: "now I see in the large group the same people that I met up close in the small group and that puts me at ease." Nevertheless, working with the group as a whole still gave rise to severe anxiety and feelings of persecution for her and she continued to treat the large group as a big, persecutory "you."

Little by little, Ronit came to meet more and more members from the large group within the small groups and these others gradually acquired individual faces and identities for her. The conductor instructed group members to change the make-up of the small groups in each session and, although Ronit and other group members sometimes voiced their opposition to this change, they eventually came to appreciate and be surprised by their acquaintance with the various group members. It should be noted that this case demonstrates the importance of constantly changing the composition of the small groups, despite potential resistance, in order to prevent the group from splitting into sub-groups. Such a split may leave members with a split-off experience, in which they feel greater intimacy and less anxiety with members they are familiar with from the small groups, while the rest remain part of the threatening, anonymous "other."

One could see how Ronit's inner turmoil gradually calmed down and how she was able to share with the group stories from her childhood about drifting about from place to place. She became more and more able to rely on the group members, rather than on the conductor, and to express her feelings of vulnerability. This was also manifest in her feeling more comfortable, free and understood in her theatrical work. She occasionally voiced feelings of dissatisfaction, but both she and the group were able to contextualize these within the framework of her personal history – which made it much easier to contain and reflect such feelings.

Ronit's process demonstrates the fact that dealing with the projection of persecutory internal objects on the group on stage is more difficult when facing the group as a whole. The division into small "playground" groups makes things easier by offering a lesser degree of projection and a greater capacity for containing the level of anxiety involved in encountering objects, which gradually become more complex and integrated for the individual. The transition between these two therapeutic setups enables little corrective experiences to cross over from the playground of the small groups to the space of the group as a whole. Ronit's case even illustrates the key role the conductor plays in the regressive processes undergone by group members. As a parent figure or a representative of parental figures, the conductor may be experienced as abandoning and neglectful; they must withstand this projection and persevere in their attempt to provide a positive alternative internalization.

This example shows how the members taking part in the therapeutic process have an opportunity to undergo a profound corrective experience through their relationship with the other group members and the conductor, as well as how important it is for the conductor to keep in mind that any progress made along this axis of visibility and acknowledgment involves internal regression. This requires the conductor to actively respond by choosing the appropriate technique on the playground-stage spectrum, the suitable level of intelligibility for the theatrical response and the kind of atmosphere they wish to foster in the group – and sometimes by answering the patient's need for a personal relationship with them. The conductor must take into account that, in such regressed states, members have a limited capacity to develop through insight and self-reflection and that their ability to tolerate and benefit from the conductor's subjectivity is similarly curtailed.

It should be noted these regressed states are often hidden, as the traumatized inner child is hiding behind the back of the functional and coherent internal adult. Lack of awareness concerning such unseen regressed states may lead to situations of pseudo-therapy and the reinforcement of the inner child's traumatic hiding behind the functional and coherent adult – keeping the patient from experiencing authenticity and spontaneity (Ogden, 1979). In this context, it is important to note that the transference relations with the conductor play a significant role in developing the capacity to integrate playfulness and visibility. The delicate emotional state of the actor, as they perform before a spectator, heightens the members' sensitivity to the conductor's real and/or imagined attitude toward the theatrical quality of their work. Any critical reaction however small – and even imagined reactions – is given considerable weight, giving rise to a lot of narcissistic vulnerability and even reviving the members' narcissistic traumas. The conductor must be well aware of this delicate state and thus of their own responses and the significance these may entail. This situation is also an opportunity for the conductor to deal with empathic failures – if these are within a reasonable scope and are handled well, they lead to both progress in the therapeutic process and the members' personal growth.

We will now present several stages that may help develop the "playground" experience and facilitate the journey toward the stage, on the path to an experience that integrates the two. Each stage is divided into sub-stages and will illustrate several techniques. The purpose of these techniques is to demonstrate how the conductor should act in order to find the emotional balance between the elements of playfulness and being visible on stage as well as the fine equilibrium with which the conductor must move and steer the group between them. We see this as our way to encourage conductors to develop and create their own exercises, which are better suited to the particular group they are conducting as well as the specific stage of its journey toward the integration of playfulness and being validated on stage.

Establishing the "playground"

Psychotherapeutic Playback Theater seeks to help group members gradually achieve the ability to playfully improvise responses to their fellow members. The initial stages of this process are characterized by fear and caution on the part of the members, who often experience the stage as threatening. Playfulness and freedom are experienced as traps which may lead to the unregulated and uncontrolled expression of shameful and anxiety-provoking parts of the self. At this stage, the goal is to help members deal with these anxieties through dramatic action. The process usually begins with a round of names, a shared physical warm-up, work in a circle and exercises that allow members to become initially acquainted with the basic situation of Psychotherapeutic Playback Theater – psychic work through the other – and its beneficial experiences. At this stage, the conductor should establish the playground experience of Psychotherapeutic Playback Theater, by working at relatively high levels of structuring (see Chapter 7) and through the utmost obfuscation of the presence of the theatrical stage.

At this initial stage, the member's experience of entering the playground should be encouraged through exercises in which each member explores themselves and only subsequently joins another member or two. This enables the space to gradually transition into a space that involves both performers and spectators (in small groups). The first course of action, at this stage, is getting members off their seats and into a structured warm-up exercise that is related to the theme of the session or the group's developmental stage. It is important for the conductor to offer simple and precise instructions, designed to reduce feelings of anxiety and not-knowing. These instructions will also orient the members toward their encounter with the theme or developmental challenge and facilitate an experience of success. At this stage, it is also important to emphasize nonverbal physical work, in which members work by themselves, to decrease the level of visibility and promote self-oriented playfulness (Winnicott, 1965). Such *warm-up exercises* can include various ways of walking around the room, exploring different physical sensations and translating these into mental images. The emphasis on movement can be followed by guided imagination, finding one's space in the room, etc.

The next stage sees the development of work in pairs and small groups. The work is relatively structured and emphasizes the principle of reflection and resonance, which is the defining principle of Psychotherapeutic Playback Theater. For example, mirroring exercises in which the essential guideline is "do like they do…" manifest the element of reflection and facilitate a simple experience of connection between members. This, in turn, leads to the potential for experiences that involve the holding of psychic material, in which one member is given a central role and is being reflected and resonated by the others. In exercises where the instruction is "do like they do…" the movement of one member becomes the movement of the other. Each member thus gains an experience of acceptance and empowerment because they are both reflected by and capable of reflecting others. The reflection of movement and sounds allows for a sense of freedom and enjoyment within a simple, clear and structured framework, in which the risk of failure is virtually non-existent. It is important to note that, while the establishment of the playground is the chief challenge facing the conductor and the group members at the initial stages of the process, it is also important to occasionally revisit it at later stages. In this gradual process, the role of the conductor is to acknowledge the fact that members are coping with the developmental challenge and to reinforce their experience of success and enjoyment in the group, seeing as playfulness is not a permanent and ongoing state, but an internal process that requires constant maintenance and cultivation (Winnicott, 1971).

As we have mentioned in various contexts before, the principle of gradualness in conducting a therapeutic process in Psychotherapeutic Playback Theater is all the more crucial in the early stages. The acceleration of this process might exacerbate feelings of shame and being at a loss, in a manner that would considerably limit playfulness over time and may even derail the entire therapeutic process.

In what follows, we will elaborate on the sub-stages leading to the establishment of the "playground" in Psychotherapeutic Playback Theater.

Physical warm-up as a driving force for theatrical work and a gateway to the playground

In most cases, the group enters the transitional space of play through a physical warm-up that corresponds to the theme of the session. This physical warm-up enables the distinction between what is defined as concrete external reality and the playful internal world. The language of physicality is the primordial language of primary infantile play and members are, in most cases, less fluent in it than in verbal language. Physical exercises and processes invite a new space of exploration, as a gateway into playfulness and creativity. When leading physical and mental warm-ups, it is important to begin with exercises that will help members experience a primary language of play and dwell on the action of playing.

At this stage, the instruction is to get off of one's chair and move about, getting one's entire body in motion. Hopefully, everyone will get up. Movement is highly significant because it encourages a transformative mindset (Ryvko, 2018). It is important for learning and change to be grounded in actual experience. The instruction is designed to lead members into theatrical work, while they are virtually unaware of it. For this to happen, one tries to make sure that the action is simultaneous and includes as many members as possible, preferably everyone. In this state, the feelings of shame and embarrassment are distributed evenly among everyone present, the element of mutual observation is limited, persecutory self-observation is alleviated and the potential for playfulness is increased. In some of the exercises in these initial stages, it is advised to add the element of having one's eyes closed, in order to further limit the extent of mutual and self-observation.

Working in a circle

After the physical warm-up, the group can transition into working in a circle. Sometimes, one can begin the session with work in a circle. This choice defines the entire group as the locus of therapeutic work and also involves a kind of nonverbal statement about the therapeutic setting (Ogden, 2003). It is likely that, when the conductor chooses to begin the process in a circle, playfulness will be rather limited at that stage and will mostly be manifest as pseudo-playfulness, which highlights executive and performative aspects in front of others. The group circle is a kind of amphitheater, which affords members a greater degree of visibility while also increasing their sense of shame and embarrassment. The situation of standing in a circle, exposed to the other members, involves feelings of discomfort and physical defenselessness. At this stage, the conductor can ask members to look at one another, nod hello and see who is there, around them. This is a simple way of structuring the members' joint affirmation and acknowledgment of the need for relatedness that is shared by everyone present.

At the following stage, the conductor can introduce unifying elements by instructing the members standing in the circle to breathe together or engage in exercises that involve an element of hand-holding, as a primary form of touch that invites attachment. The use of the circle stresses the gradually coalescing "groupness" and the desire for unity and attachment, namely, the vital components of the initial stages of the process. According to Jung (2003), the circle is even imbued with the archetypal themes of the distinction between inside and outside, sacred and profane, thus offering a symbolic representation of the transformative space of the group and the community while simultaneously being the most primordial symbol of the self.

We will now introduce three circle-based practice techniques that facilitate the transition from the playground to the stage.

Word and motion in the circle

Each member is asked, in turn, to express how they feel in the present moment, using sound and movement. Sound and movement are the most primary and primitive elements of theatrical work. Utilizing the elements of movement and sound causes exhalation with every action, increasing sensations of relaxation and release on a physiological level. Once the member has created such a sound-and-movement expression, the other members reflect it back to them. Later in the process, this exercise can be directed more openly, shifting the group's response from reflection to resonance – meaning, from trying to copy the original as precisely as possible to an attempt to offer a more interpretive, subjective and metaphoric expression of the experience the observer has perceived. In this setup, the entire group takes a moment to look at a single member and the experience of emergence may arise for an instant.

This primary exercise creates a group resonance, which borrows theatrical elements into the playground and thus helps members move toward its integration with the stage. The theatrical piece comprises a sequence of actions, which amount to a dramatic event. In this exercise, actions join each other and complete one another, forming a primary and harmonious group creation. This grants members an experience of theatrical aesthetics characteristic of dramatic work, whose potential enjoyment they can now experience in the playground, without having to go on stage. At the group level, this simple exercise includes elements of listening, accepting the other and a nascent attempt at reflection processes – elements which are the cornerstones of the therapeutic process in Psychotherapeutic Playback Theater.

From the perspective of the group members, this initial and simple exercise already confronts them with the developmental challenge of being playful under the gaze of others. Therefore, one should expect a decrease in playfulness, meaning that most members will try to maintain a relatively familiar, limited and safe space. For this reason, they will move and make sounds in a manner that is similar to those who went before them, with slight alterations and a general air of awkwardness. The conductor should encourage members to find their own unique voice and express it fully. It is crucial that the conductor's promptings at this stage are as positive as possible, offering accepting and empathic feedback on the members' limited playfulness. Being critical might increase persecutory self-observation and curtail playfulness even further. Reflective interpretations should be used very sparingly, at best, during this stage. If the conductor still decides to offer an interpretation regarding the use of imitation and repetition as ways of keeping anxiety at bay, it is important that they do so in a way that normalizes and universalizes this phenomenon. In addition, they should point out the instances of difference within the abovementioned similarity, in order to support such differences without being judgmental toward their limited playfulness. It is recommended that this reflection serve to legitimize imitation as a way of reducing performance anxiety. Such acceptance may later lead to greater playfulness, given that Psychotherapeutic Playback Theater utilizes this manner of imitation in later stages of its process as well.

Object transformation in the circle

The conductor holds an imaginary ball in his hand and passes it to the members, who pass it among themselves. Each time a member gets the imaginary ball, they play with it a little and it grows bigger. In this manner, the ball is passed between the members until it becomes too big for one person to handle and two members must hold it together. The members keep passing the ball and the ball continues to grow, requiring more and more members to hold it each time. By the end of the process, the ball has become so huge that it is held by the entire group. This exercise simulates and prefigures the group's future developmental stages and the development of its capacity for shared holding. The metaphor inherent in this exercise indicates the mutual relevance and even interdependence of the group members in the therapeutic process of Psychotherapeutic Playback Theater.

Leaning back in the circle

Much like the previous exercise, this one also highlights and simulates shared holding. When standing in a circle, group members are instructed to look in each other's eyes. They are then invited to hold hands in the circle, so that each member can put his weight on the other member. This exercise demonstrates and simulates group holding and containment and the creation of an integral structure as a container.

Working in pairs

After working in a circle, the group can transition to working in pairs. This mode of work is designed to encourage interpersonal interactions through action in the interpersonal playground. Dividing the group into pairs could be likened to a swing in an actual playground: both sides choose to get on the swing; both must feel and understand the way the ride works and act by shifting the balance and changing positions back and forth. It is important for any instructions given at this stage to be elaborate and clear, so as to supply a steady foundation for spontaneity, playfulness and mutuality and allow members to be free of overly conscious thinking. It is important to consider that this situation involves a high potential for embarrassment because of the intimacy it creates. As a way of dealing with this feeling of embarrassment and fostering a sense of intimacy, Psychotherapeutic Playback Theater offers active engagement in the shared playful task. The process of play even facilitates a shared holding of embarrassment. In addition, the playful and dramatic tasks entail metaphoric thinking about content and process.

The goal of pair-based exercises is to establish dramatic actions through simple exercises that are based on clear instructions and that contain an element of imitation. The simplicity of these exercises is designed to minimize, as much as possible, the possibility of failure – which increases the members' feeling of success and their potential for taking part in the creation of a shared, positive dyad. These exercises involve elements of physicality, mutual play and shared movement. In addition, they entail the element of the predefined roles of leader and follower, which facilitates the exploration and discovery of and experimentation with leading and following and supports the ability to alternate smoothly between these two roles. The roles of leader and follower and the uniform transition back and forth between the two are some of the fundamental components of improvisation. In addition, these exercises express and allow members to experience the dilemma of self-other relations and the requisite oscillation between dominance and subservience in these relations, as it is manifest in the act of improvisation.

The mirror technique

The group is divided into pairs and the members in each pair stand facing each other. At first, one of them leads with a certain movement and the other follows as their mirror, imitating their movement as accurately as possible. The instruction is to move together in a synchronized motion, like in a mirror, so that an external observer would not be able to tell which one is leading and which one is following. Then, the two members switch roles. The conductor asks the pairs to switch roles several more times, until they begin moving together without assigning leader and follower. At this point, the two members of each pair are changing roles spontaneously, creating synchronized movement that is grounded in both nonverbal communication and shared creation.

The camera technique

The group is divided into pairs, with one member standing in front and the other standing behind them. The person in front is defined as the "camera," while the one behind is defined as the "photographer." The camera-member stands with their eyes closed, while the photographer-member leads them around the room. Once the photographer has found the picture they want to take – some object that they want to focus on and show the camera-member – they carefully aim the "camera" to face this object and then give them a little "click" on the shoulder. The camera opens their eyes and immediately closes them, just like a camera's shutter. Each "photographer" takes five pictures and then the two members switch roles. After both have played both roles, they share which pictures were meaningful to them and talk about their experience throughout this process.

Exploring spaces in pairs

The group is divided into pairs and music is played in the background. One member in each pair forms a sculpture, while the other explores the spaces created by this sculpture, moving around them and through these spaces. This exploration can be done with one's arms, legs, elbows, head, etc. After a few minutes, the conductor asks each pair to switch roles. After switching roles several more times, the conductor asks the members to keep exploring the spaces, but to do so simultaneously – resulting in a shared dance.

After the possibility of working in the interpersonal space of the pair has been established, the group's playfulness space can be expanded by joining pairs together and creating groups of four and, later on, groups of eight. Thus, for example, one can join two pairs that are mirroring each other and form a group of four and then take two such groups of four and form a group of eight that is engaged in the mirror game. The greater the number of members taking part in shared work, the more the playing space is established and expanded in a bigger and more complex group.

Working in groups of three or four

Working in groups of three or four allows members to work with stories, which are the foundation of Psychotherapeutic Playback Theater, and to create theatrical images in response to these stories. In the small group, one member shares a story and the other two or three members create a theatrical improvisation in response to it.

Work in small groups in the playground of Psychotherapeutic Playback Theater facilitates a moving process, which creates, in a short amount of time, "domes" of intimacy throughout the room, which envelop the small groups that are working simultaneously. In this process, the members of each group are deeply focused on each other and each movement, no matter how slight, is given meaning. One can begin to sense the emergence of a space that is "ours," of an experience of "we-ness"; this is because the piece created through theatrical response belongs neither to the teller nor to the playing members, but is the result of shared creation. Here are two emblematic techniques for work in groups of three:

From word and image to scene

The group is divided into groups of three: one member tells a story and the other two listen. Each of the listeners chooses a word or an image from the story that they find crucial to understanding it. The first member creates a movement that offers an emotional expression of their chosen word or image. After the movement is over, they freeze to form a sculpture, which should express the emotional state they believe the story embodies. As they freeze, they also utter the chosen word. The second member joins in and does the same: they, too, move in accordance with their chosen word, freeze into a sculpture that is an emotional expression of this word and, finally, say this word out loud. Once the two sculptures are frozen side by side, they hold this freeze for five seconds and then shift into a movement dialogue, which develops into a freely improvised scene, with the chosen word echoing in the background. After the two members have finished their theatrical response, they return to the teller and listen to their thoughts and feelings about the scene they have played, making sure to check if the teller would like an additional theatrical response.

Teller, sculpture, sculptor

The members move about the room to music, doing a movement warm-up that involves stretching and making circles with various parts of the body. They are gradually asked to see which story comes to their mind while they are warming up. The conductor stresses that the definition of "story" is very broad and may include virtually any content – dreams, wishes, feelings, etc. Members are asked to make this story as detailed as possible in their mind – fleshing out the characters, physical experience, place, time, smells, colors, tastes and so on. This part of the exercise can serve to give rise to stories and flesh them out within any session plan.

Members then form groups of three and are advised to pick members they are less acquainted with as their partners. One of the three members is the "teller," who shares a short story with the other two. The second member is the "sculpture," who is modified by the third member, the "sculptor." The sculptor sculpts the sculpture by positioning them in three different positions or sculptures, which correspond to the beginning, middle and end of the story. The story can be carved out in any way: according to the narrative shared, the teller's emotional state, a single evolving metaphor, three different metaphors, etc. The teller can ask to modify the sculptures to make them more accurate and the sculptor performs the necessary corrections.

Once the sculptor has finished creating all three sculptures, the sculpture-member connects the three of these into a sequence of motion, a movement-phrase, and they are also allowed to add their own movements between each sculpted position as well as after the final position. Once the exercise is over, the members briefly share their experiences. They repeat the exercise three times, so that each member can experience each of the three roles. They will thus each perform a movement-phrase as a fluid sculpture, which is based on the story as well as the positions determined by the two other members. This phrase could serve the member during the "Putting the Playground on Stage" technique, which will be presented shortly.

While this technique seems simple, it contains a significant core of the principles on which Psychotherapeutic Playback Theater is founded. It demonstrates the creation of a shared group playing space and the setting up of shared creation in a short amount of time. Members often report that it quickly establishes an experience of closeness and intimacy. Furthermore, it illustrates the sequence of deconstructing, refining, exploring and then reintegrating each element, which is characteristic of Psychotherapeutic Playback Theater.

This technique can also be practiced in pairs, by combining the roles of "sculpture" and "sculptor" – the sculptor sculpts themselves into beginning, middle and end statues, the teller makes their adjustments and, at the end, the sculptor/sculpture creates the movement sequence.

Putting the Playground on Stage – Using Movement-Phrases to Build a Theatrical Performance (continuing the "Teller, Sculpture, Sculptor" technique)

This sequence involves a shift from the playing space of the small groups to the playing space of the entire group – a space that has more stage-like qualities and entails a greater level of visibility. This shift is designed to help members experience emergence within the structured transition from the playing space of the small groups to that of the entire group. This transition is achieved by combining each member's movement-phrase, which they created by drawing on the story and the movements of other members, into shared work on stage. In this version, when the sculpture creates their movement-phrase, they repeat it several times so that they know it by heart. Additionally, once the work done in groups of three is over, the conductor may choose to instruct the members to spread out across the room and continue exploring their movement-phrase.

The conductor then explains the rules for the transition to working on stage – each member enters the group playing space with their movement-phrase, which they repeat wholeheartedly, while noticing their location on stage in relation to the other members. It is also possible to create a dialogue between movement-phrases. The members begin their movement work immediately after getting up from their seat and only end it once they have sat back down. One can enter the group playing space only when the teller of the story, on which this phrase is based, is sitting in the audience. Members can enter the group playing space several times, as instructed by the conductor. We have found that the instruction to enter the group playing space at least three times is useful, as it allows members to deal with the anxiety of the first attempt and frees them up to engage in the ensuing dialogues between movement-phrases.

It is important that the entire duration of the work in the group playing space is accompanied by background music that is sufficiently prominent. The musical envelope serves as a kind of "musical container" for what is happening. We have found that music that has psychedelic elements can be very efficient in helping members access their internal world and shift to primary thinking and surreal theatrical aesthetics. We have also found that shifting back and forth between strong and swelling music and minor and somewhat elegiac music is valuable: such oscillation allows stories with different emotional flavors to surface in the group playing space. The changing music creates a certain improvisational space through the encounter between a movement-phrase that has one emotional shade and background music that has another emotional shade.

This technique helps members bring the playground on stage by working in a partially structured space, which may lower their level of anxiety. This enables the exploration of a piece of art that has been created in response to the emotional material of another person – demonstrating the principle of expanding the self through the other, a key principle of Psychotherapeutic Playback Theater. This practice facilitates exposure to the space which opens precisely through one's willingness to work for the other and invites new experiences. In this instance, members have experiences both within the aesthetic container and in front of it, by exploring where to situate their movement-phrase in relation to those of the other members on stage. This results in a product that achieves considerable aesthetic and artistic value in a relatively short time and by working within a structured space. This experience increases the members' level of confidence in their theatrical abilities, in preparation for on stage work in Psychotherapeutic Playback Theater.

On stage

After having practiced the playground with the group, we are ready to work on stage, in various styles, at different levels of structuration and in accordance with the group's developmental stage. It should be noted that once theatrical response on stage has become available, it must be maintained through warm-up exercises, the combination of working in small groups and with the entire group and the application of different levels of structuration, as discussed in the following chapter.

In conclusion, the process of Psychotherapeutic Playback Theater seeks to develop playfulness, creativity and spontaneity in the group's "here and now" space and, eventually, allowing members to experience such playfulness on stage. This process facilitates the emergence of diverse aspects of the self in the group space. Through a flexible and creative process, group members explore and express psychic material in front of supportive and empathic others. This process is vital to the development of the self. In the next chapter, we will discuss the different ways of introducing psychic material in the group's stage space, by using forms of structuration that are adapted to the different stages of the process.

Chapter 7

Such stuff as containers are made on

Levels of structuring in Psychotherapeutic Playback Theater

Ronen Kowalsky, Nir Raz, Shoshi Keisari

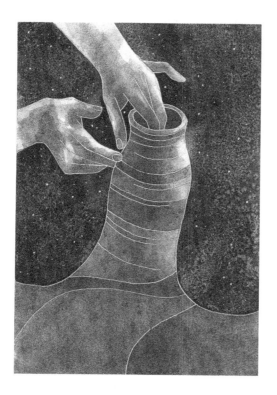

Figure 7.1

Rooted as it is in aesthetic traditions, Psychotherapeutic Playback Theater relies on theatrical images, movement and music. These elements create a dialogue between the narrator and the theatrical response as an aesthetic form which organizes psychic material and elaborates the story and creates

DOI: 10.4324/9781003167822-8

a container for introducing insight and exploring new meanings and perspectives (Rowe, 2007).

The metaphoric concept of the container, as presented by Bion (1963), is an apt illustration of the way Psychotherapeutic Playback Theater structures psychic material as a significant tool in therapy. The role of the container is to link primary psychic experiences and imbue them with meaning or, in Bion's words, "to make the unthinkable thinkable." In Psychotherapeutic Playback Theater, the visible theatrical response expresses the personal narrative and creates a container for the primary materials of psychic experience. Dramatic metaphors organize the psychic material derived from the story and allow the client to encounter and work through them. As a container for the story, the aesthetic patterns of Playback Theater restructure personal experience, imbuing the story with the potential for new meaning.

In developing the concept of the container, Bion (ibid.) drew his ideas from philosopher Immanuel Kant (1998), who argued that intuition without concept is blind and that concept without intuition is empty. This serves as the foundation for our view of the theatrical pattern as capable of containing intuitive psychic material within aesthetic concepts that are charged with meaning. Bion conceptualized this process in terms of beta-elements (β) and alpha-function (α). Beta-elements represent raw sensory material, pure data that is unlinked and void of any meaning stemming from such raw material. The alpha-function is the activity that collects and brings together a cluster of beta-elements and provides them with a shared meaning. The alpha-function is the activity represented in the role of the container (thus the use of the term "function," which is borrowed from the field of mathematics and which represents action), while beta-elements represent raw material, which is only given meaning when contained within the container (the alpha-function) and which remains meaningless when it is outside of that container. Bion describes the relationship between the alpha-function and beta-elements, between container and contained, as a dynamic one. Containment creates meaning for certain beta-elements, but leaves other beta-elements outside of it. Moreover, one of the consequences of a good-enough container is the creation of new beta-elements outside of it. This process challenges the container and may result in one of three potential reactions.

i   The disintegration of the container and the dispersal of beta-elements – the response to a situation in which raw psychic material (beta-elements) are created outside the container is the disintegration of the container and the dispersal of beta-elements, raw psychic material, across an ungraspable and meaningless space. For example, this may occur when the conductor has given up on finding meaning in the material brought up by the group, thus, in fact, abandoning his role. In this situation, theatrical response fails to hold the psychic material arising from the story and the experience is one of meaningless and unintelligible theatrical chaos.

ii A rigid container – rigidly insisting on a particular container, despite the emergence of new psychic material which is left outside of it, accelerates the emergence of new beta-elements outside the container, draining it of meaning. For example, this happens when the conductor repeatedly insists on imbuing the new material introduced by the group with particular meaning. Although this meaning was adequate when it was first presented, the conductor's insistence accelerates the process by which it becomes irrelevant for the group. Theatrically, this is manifest in the insistence on certain structured forms and theatrical aesthetics which are increasingly experienced as limiting creativity, as inauthentic and especially as precluding the introduction of new material and its exploration in a creative space, in a way that facilitates the discovery of new insight.

iii A flexible container – the conductor leads the group in a process of leaving established meaning behind and looking for new meaning that could integrate and contain new psychic material, which then joins existing material. In fact, this situation is the desired response, because it promotes development, instead of hindering it, as the previous two responses do. Nevertheless, it requires both the members and the conductor to tolerate a certain amount of anxiety. This is because it depends on one being in a mental state that Bion (1967) calls "preconception": a temporary absence of meaning while one is in the process of seeking it out. The container thus described is a flexible one, one which adapts itself to the emerging contents and the group process. On the theatrical level, this state is manifest in the flexible transition between different theatrical forms and between the adoption and relinquishment of a particular aesthetic. It is assumed that members are temporarily capable of tolerating a lack of certainty and meaning while improvising as a way of creating space for the introduction of new contents and revelations – as mentioned, this situation involves a certain degree of anxiety. The flexible reaction is therapeutically significant because it helps members contain these temporary experiences of anxiety, not-understanding and meaninglessness, seeing as such containment is crucial, according to Bion, for true psychic development.

One can define and characterize a spectrum of different setups of Psychotherapeutic Playback Theater according to their level of structuring (Kowalsky et al., 2019). This spectrum can be very useful for the conductor in their attempt to find the particular setup that is most relevant to the populations comprising the group and the group's present stage in the therapeutic process. The level of structuring in the therapeutic process and in the creative process is constantly reevaluated in accordance with the needs of the group and the process. In addition, the structuring spectrum is a significant conceptual tool that helps adapt Psychotherapeutic Playback Theater to different populations. One can pinpoint where the group population is located on the spectrum in terms of the level of structuring it currently has (over-structuring or under-structuring) and the level of structuring it requires.

Our experience has taught us that members belonging to certain populations can be characterized as being in a state of under-structuring and in need of structuring as part of the therapeutic process. For some, this is an inherent characteristic of the illness with which they are dealing, such as members diagnosed with schizophrenia, depression or disorders involving psychotic or depressive states. Members belonging to other populations can be characterized as dealing with temporary under-structuring, such as members coping with traumatic situations, undergoing substance abuse rehabilitation or struggling with emotionally challenging transitions including immigration, divorce, chronic or terminal physical illness, etc. Other populations which require structuring as part of the therapeutic process are those whose experience in Psychotherapeutic Playback Theater confronts them with a fundamental difficulty with empathy and understanding the other. This category includes members diagnosed on the autism spectrum or those suffering from manic states or various personality disorders. In contrast, populations that are in a state of over-structuring include, for example, members who are mental health professionals. It is important to note that these characterizations merely provide a general guideline and that the conductor must carefully evaluate the particular group they are working with, at each particular time period. One should take into account that there is sometimes an intricate relationship between over-structuring and under-structuring. For example, when over-structuring is used as a defense against the experience of breakdown, this requires the conductor to move flexibly back and forth along the structuring axis, in accordance with the state of the group at each particular moment.

Figure 7.2 illustrates the level of structuring spectrum, which facilitates the integration of the different elements within the theatrical work (Kowalsky et al., 2019): one side of the spectrum represents a high level of structuring, achieved through the use of structured theatrical patterns, which organize psychic material and actively imbue it with meaning; the other side of the spectrum represents a relatively low level of structuring and greater freedom in the theatrical response, whereby members react to psychic material and represent its various aspects with considerable creative license, without pre-planning or a pre-determined theatrical pattern.

The common course of development for a Psychotherapeutic Playback Theater group traces a shift from relatively structured patterns to open patterns, with a relatively low level of structuring. Naturally, in the initial stages of the process, the group exhibits a greater need for higher levels of structuring, for a tight container which is manifest in improvising within pre-structured and familiar theatrical patterns and improvisations which

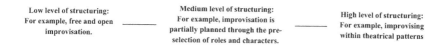

| Low level of structuring: For example, free and open improvisation. | Medium level of structuring: For example, improvisation is partially planned through the pre-selection of roles and characters. | High level of structuring: For example, improvising within theatrical patterns |

Figure 7.2 The level of structuring spectrum.

tend more toward the realistic and the concrete. However, when the group comprises populations with a tendency for over-structuring, it is important to strive for open forms even in the initial stages of the work, to balance out this predilection.

The role of the conductor is to gauge, at each stage of the group process, its condition and the level of structuring required. The more the group is suffering from under-structuring and the more chaotic and disorganized psychic material tends to surface in an anxiety-provoking manner, the greater the need for a higher level of structuring in the group and creative processes that would gather these materials into a meaning-making container. In the spirit of Kant and Bion, this state can be conceptualized as one of *under-containment*: "intuitions without concepts are blind," according to Kant (1998); beta-elements floating in space, yearning for an alpha-function that would contain them and imbue them with meaning, according to Bion (1963). In this state, one can resort to several methods for raising the level of structuring, such as the use of structured theatrical forms, pre-selecting playing members to the theatrical response, having the tellers cast playing members as characters from their story, assigning a fixed seat for the teller next to the conductor, instructing the teller to give their story a title, observing the clear and fixed ritual and structure of the session and carefully recapitulating what is going on in the process several times throughout the session.

Daria, a 28-year-old woman, talks about her role in a groundbreaking education project. As one of the founders of this project, in the past three years, she had a key position with a considerable degree of authority. She had found her work very satisfying and meaningful and seemed to be able to express her skills. She was very successful and felt that she had found her place professionally. The project did very well and began expanding and, the more it grew, the more its original staff had to bring in new people and create new positions of authority. Daria was required to consign some of her authorities to new figures who joined the organization. At some point, she described that certain aspects of her position were reassigned to other people and she now had to discuss and wait for approval on subjects which were once her prerogative. Daria depicted the difficulties this change entailed, her experience that her place has been undermined and the distress and anxiety she has been feeling lately, following all these transitions. It was very difficult for her to adapt to this new reality.

The playing members presented a movement-based theatrical response, which began with one actor working into the playing space, aesthetically arranging chairs and cloths as a work of art, with music playing in the background. The look on her face was radiant, passionate and full of creative intent. Her movements were a light, free dance. She then walked to the end of the playing space and gazed at her creation from afar. At this point, other playing members started entering the playing space, walking around the installation she had created and looking at it, also seeming to examine her work of art. Next, they began taking the chairs and the cloths that made up the installation and moving them from about, spreading the cloths on the floor, stacking the chairs. This activity took a long time and served as a central part of the theatrical response, manifesting in the playing space the chaos and dissolution of something that initially felt complete and finalized. The actor who played Daria walked around the circumference of the splaying space, looking helplessly on at what was happening. She said: "what's going on here? This isn't supposed to be this way."

After the theatrical response was concluded, Daria said: "when I saw the improvisation, I couldn't understand what you were doing and I just disconnected. Something about it made me angry. It seemed unrelated to my story, I got lost." Daria's response can be seen to indicate her experience that her story was "under-contained" by the reflection, because the latter used an open, abstract and relatively distanced form. In the theatrical reflection, the playing members tried to introduce several significant elements from the story into the playing space and show a narrative axis that connects them. However, their use of an abstract dramatic idiom, which involved movement with virtually no text, meant that the teller was unable to recognize her story in the dramatic reflection. Daria's story concerns a present theme from her life and one which has not yet been worked through; it therefore gives rise to a high level of anxiety. In this situation, it seems that Daria and the group need a more structured process and a tighter container. Responding to this need, the conductor and the group chose to work with a more structured form, by pre-assigning several roles from the story – the teller, a figure which represents the educational project itself and various people who came to work on the project. The group members chose to work via the structured pattern of "interrupted monologues," in which each character delivers several lines of monologue and is then interrupted by another character. This pattern gives each character room to express themselves separately, eventually creating a structured image that is imbued with several perspectives about the situation, while the repeated interruptions emphasize the conflict between the different characters. In response to this second reflection, Daria said:

> I felt that, in the second one, I could recognize my story and myself. I was more able to see the complexity of my story – it wasn't only about feeling lonely and helpless, but also about choosing my partners in this project. Through the monologues of my character and the character of

the project's representation, I could also see my success and the way the project was expanding, my desire to try and adapt to the situation and overcome this difficulty and the hope that, although this kind of adaptation is painful, it is still possible.

In contrast, some groups will feel stifled within overly tight containers. They will experience such containers as limiting their emotional expression and their creativity and as repeatedly leading them to the same banal insights. This condition can be termed *over-containment*: "concepts without intuition are empty," according to Kant (1998); a rigid container that is evacuating beta-elements, according to Bion (1963). Over-containment is a state in which old meaning is forced on new material in an excessively rigid manner, to the extent that development is curtailed. In such states, one should resort to less structured theatrical patterns, such as free improvisation, without pre-selecting or casting playing members; the story should not be given a title, the teller can be allowed to tell their story from wherever they are sitting in the group, one can occasionally alter the ritual and the setting, engage in fewer, shorter or more abstract recapitulations, or forgo recapitulation entirely in favor of dwelling in the experience itself.

In a Psychotherapeutic Playback Theater group, 36-year-old Jason shared a story about his complicated relationship with his younger brother. Jason described a very loving relationship between him and his brother, alongside feelings of envy and a sense that his parents somewhat favor his brother over him. Over the years, his brother had suffered from developmental difficulties, which forced the parents to step up and care for him more substantially as well as to be very lenient with him, while always being strict and demanding with Jason. Jason described having many arguments with his brother recently, sharing that he felt impatient with his brother, that he had a "short fuse," as if everything his brother said or did made him angry. The conductor asked Jason to give examples of sentences that he said to his brother and that his brother said to him. He then asked Jason to pick two members to play himself and his brother. Once in the playing space, the playing members engaged in a dialogue that was based on the sentences Jason shared during the interview phase. Later on, each line of dialogue led the playing members to throw a piece of cloth at each other, as an expression of the anger and frustration of the two brothers and their sense of weariness and exasperation at their ongoing quarrel. The scene ended with each brother accusing the other to their face, until both playing members "dropped" the scene and walked off the playing space, each in a different direction. Once the theatrical response was over, the conductor turned back to Jason, who said: "I want to thank the players, they really showed me the conflict, but I feel that there was something missing here and I can't say what."

It appeared that the playing members' exclusive focus on the conflict between the two brothers made the theatrical container all too rigid, only addressed a single aspect of the story and did not facilitate better holding of the intricacies of the teller's experience. This situation left many aspects of his subjective experience outside of the theatrical container, including the brothers' loving relationship, the younger brother's vulnerability, the parents' concern for his future and Jason's professional success, which he secured through his parents' expectations of him. In response to Jason's words, the conductor suggested that the group should perform once again, inviting them to engage in an open theatrical improvisation. One by one, the members came up from the audience and entered the open playing space. They introduced different voices and many more aspects of the story, from their own subjective perspectives and their personal encounters with the story's contents. One member came into the playing space and gave a monologue that held the perspective of the younger brother, who looks up to his older brother; two others came into the playing space together and, through movement work in the corner of the room, created a children's game in which the older brother taught the younger brother how to assemble an airplane; the two playing members from the first theatrical response took the playing space again, once more presenting the conflict between the brothers and the sentences Jason gave during the interview; yet another member positioned herself in another corner and represented the voice of the mother, who talked about her two sons and their relationship; finally, one player put a chair next to a table and pretended to be climbing up, while another player sat down on the floor, looking at him from below and eagerly applauding him. It seemed that Jason was very moved by the new theatrical response, reacting to certain moments with a broad smile. After it was over, he said with glistening eyes:

> there were some incredibly moving things here, things I did even talk about, that reminded me of feelings I had forgotten in my relationship with my brother, things that it felt good to remember. This has given me some things to think about.

It seems that the multiple perspectives enabled by the open improvisation allowed a more complex and complete experience to surface, the kind of experience that may lead to new insight, as an opportunity for change.

According to Bion (1963), a *"good-enough" container function* will allow new primary material to emerge outside of it and thus promote the development of thinking and creativity. However, in many cases and as a natural part of the therapeutic process, there are states of over-containment or under-containment, as mentioned above: over-containment involves the forcing of old meaning onto new material in an excessively rigid manner that hinders development; under-containment involves primary psychic material being left floating in space, without being given any meaning whatsoever. From Bion's perspective (ibid.), development appears as a process in which one oscillates between creating a shared meaning and relinquishing this meaning so that new primary material can emerge, which in turn is given new meaning, which will eventually be relinquished to facilitate the emergence of new primary material and so forth. It is, therefore, important for the conductor to evaluate the group process at each and every stage and adjust the level of structuring informing the theatrical response in order to establish a container that is better adapted to the group's needs. When the conductor insists on forcing a particular idea or acts at a level of structuring that is ill-adapted to the group process, this may lead to the emergence of resistance or rebellion, at best, or to the members placating the conductor and the container growing ever emptier, at worst. On the one hand, the conductor may force their idea, thus creating a container that is ill-adapted to the group and that will therefore remain empty; on the other hand, they may give up on their idea entirely, leaving the group blind, not knowing how to process, devoid of any idea that could achieve meaning.

The aim is for the conductor to think on their feet, to identify group voices and create an appropriately flexible container that will be able to contain these voices and imbue them with meaning; meanwhile, they should also leave room for additional voices to emerge and be witnessed outside of this container, leading to the creation of new containers. Thus, the group container is established anew each time. The two vignettes presented above show the manner in which the conductor must constantly examine how the different patterns are being played with, while continuously seeking to adapt the density of the container's substance to the group. Exploring the structuring level of the work being done in Psychotherapeutic Playback Theater in light of Bion's (1963) thinking may lead to its conceptualization as the (paraphrasing Shakespeare) "stuff as containers are made on." At higher levels of structuring, the container can be viewed as made of a material that is more rigid and tight-fitting in relation to the psychic material it contains; while at lower levels of structuring, one can picture the container as made of a more flexible substance.

Structured setups for theatrical response

In the early stages of the group process, the conductor structures the ritual and uses it to establish a clear setting. The ritual defines a sequence of fixed occurrences, within which there is also room for creative freedom. The ritual begins with warm-up exercises that entail physical, mental and interactive elements, after which members take their seats in a semi-circle facing the playing space. At this stage, one can have a *check-in round*, which can also include brief dramatic responses in response to emerging material; next, the group can be divided into smaller work groups, in order to establish the *playground* experience; then, the conductor should recap the experiences of the small groups in the large group; then, the conductor will ask who wants to volunteer to be the teller. The teller will come and sit in the chair next to the conductor. The teller's seat is always next to the conductor's, facing the playing space, at the center of the semi-circle. This location represents the key role of the teller and the attunement of the playing members to them. The adjacent presence of the conductor represents the conductor's role of keeping the teller safe and providing an envelope for the teller and the process, given the teller's sensitive position after having entrusted their story to the other members. In later stages of the group process, some of the steps of this ritual can become more flexible. For example, the conductor can allow the teller to share their story from wherever they happen to be sitting. The conductor will choose this option when they feel that the group is providing sufficient mental holding for the teller and that having the teller sit next to them may be perceived as regression from more advanced group relations to a dyadic relationship and as encouraging a degree of dependence on the conductor that is inappropriate of the group's present stage of development.

Structuring, first and foremost, means the degree to which dramatic work is structured. Structuring often comprises three stages: (1) dividing the contents of the story into several distinct elements; (2) developing a tangible theatrical representation for each element separately; (3) integrating the various elements to create a new, harmonious piece, which holds all the elements together and facilitates transitions between them.

The integration of the different elements can be done through various means, which represent different psychic actions. The use of structuring in Psychotherapeutic Playback Theater must address two kinds of containers – the aesthetic container and the narrative container. The *aesthetic container* gives psychic material meaning by organizing it within a theatrical pattern, which evokes an aesthetic experience in the spectator. The pattern includes such aspects as the use of space, color, movement, music, etc. The establishment of this container reserves a special place for the dramatic composition or mise-en-scène and its respective aspects of space and form. The aesthetic container gives stimuli new experiential meaning and plays a considerable role in making the unthinkable thinkable or, in Bion's (1978) words, "this aesthetic element of beauty makes a very difficult situation tolerable." The *narrative container* organizes the contents of the narrative sequence in a way that grants them new meaning. This organization can be chronological or thematic, while the latter may also draw on various theoretical conceptualizations.

These two containers exist simultaneously in every therapeutic action, in the sense that the aesthetic container has narrative meaning and the narrative container has aesthetic meaning. In this sense, one can view any action in the therapeutic space – whether dramatic or verbal; whether it is an act of interpretation, mirroring or intervention – as simultaneously involving both narrative and aesthetic structuring. It is important to note that both the aesthetic and the narrative containers can succumb to states of over- and under-structuring and that the conductor must look for the level of structuring suitable to the group at each and every stage for both these aspects.

The following sections address the different levels at which the theatrical response can be structured and the manner in which these levels offer different degrees of density for the aesthetic and narrative containers.

Structured theatrical patterns as a container for theatrical response

At stages and in situations which require a high level of structuring, the conductor instructs the members to contain the theatrical response within pre-structured theatrical patterns. This instruction may include the theatrical response done in small groups; the theatrical responses during the check-in round and the theatrical response in the theater improvisation performed in front of the entire group.

The structuring of the theatrical pattern can involve three dimensions: space, time and contents. These dimensions are not entirely separate and, in most cases, the structuring affects more than one dimension at the same time. For example, structuring in space often entails the structuring of contents and the structuring of contents is often manifest in a structured use of space. In this section, we will demonstrate various structuring possibilities through several pre-determined patterns for improvising in Playback Theater. These patterns, known as "short forms," were developed by the founder of Playback Theater, Jonathan Fox (Rowe, 2007). The use of additional structured patterns is further demonstrated in Chapters 4 and 8.

Spatial structuring

This type of structuring is performed through the organization of the various elements arising from the contents of the story according to their location in the playing space. The *arrowhead* pattern, for example, is a pattern that structures the theatrical response according to a spatial logic. In this pattern, one of the playing members is closer to the front of the playing space, while the other two playing members are further away, standing toward the back. This creates an arrowhead shape or "narrative V." Similarly, another structural-theatrical pattern can be used to determine that some of the psychic elements of the story will be presented downstage, while other psychic elements will be given room upstage. An example of such a pattern is taken from the case of Chen, a 28-year-old man who shares his decision to wait yet another year before resuming his academic studies. He talks about how interested he is in that particular field of study and lists the rational reasons behind his decision that now is not the right time. Later on, he recalls certain negative experiences from his past years as a student suffering from an attention deficit disorder and learning difficulties. He finishes his story by saying that, after he had made the decision, he felt a heavy weight being lifted from his shoulders. Three members entered the playing space and arranged themselves in the "arrowhead" structure. The member standing at the point of the arrowhead, which represents the more explicit voices, expressed the feeling of relief that accompanied the decision and repeated the rational motives Chen mentioned. Then, the second member, standing behind him (at the upstage) and to his right, expressed fear of failure at the prospect of going back to school. He brought up experiences of frustration and despair from Chen's scholarly past. Then, the third member, who was also standing behind the arrow-head-member and beside the second member, in the left side of the arrow, expressed an interest in and desire toward the chosen field of study. He also voiced an experience of knowledge, curiosity and success as well as a sense of optimism about Chen's engagement with this field. The simultaneous presence of these three voices together on a single playing space enables the integration of these different experiences. Positioning the second and third voices more upstage indicates that these are more implicit voices and that they involve a greater degree of interpretation on the part of the playing members. This illustrates the manner in which the spatial structuring of the theatrical response also entails a structuring of contents. After the theatrical response was over, Chen said, "well, you figured out that it's not that simple…" He then told the group about how lonely he felt about the discrepancies in his experience as a student, between his sense of knowledge, understanding and even being interested in the material and repeatedly failing his tests. What Chen had shared inspired other members to share about gaps in their own self-image, in relation to confusing experiences in which success and failure were coupled in a contradictory way.

The emotional elements of a story can also be given equal room, either by positioning them in the same space or by emphasizing their contrast through a "partition" of the playing space into distinct and separate locations. For example, the *talking heads* pattern affords all the inner voices of the story an equal place: four members stand in a line, each of them portraying a different inner voice. All these voices have the same status in the playing space, both in relation to each other and in relation to positions of the teller and the audience. In addition, each inner voice has their own separate location. This diversifies the perspectives in the story. In turn, each member delivers a monologue representing their respective inner voice, until another member begins a monologue for a different voice, interrupting the previous one. When necessary, the conductor may utilize additional interventions, such as having the different voices engage in a dialogue or having them move up or down the playing space, in order to represent the heightening or weakening of a certain voice and its transition into conscious emotional experience or its retreat into unconscious experience.

Ravit, a 43-year-old woman, shared a story about a trip to Romania that she took with her nuclear family, to explore their family history. One evening, on their way back to the hotel after dining in a restaurant, Ravit noticed an abandoned synagogue and, next to it, a faded memorial plaque mentioning the local Jewish community, which had been murdered in the Second World War. Ravit was overcome by sadness, curiosity and an unexplained longing, and wanted to go inside. Her children were against it, saying that they were already tired and did not have the energy "for more of this holocaust dejection." Ravit's husband sided with their children, saying that "there's no choice. They're tired and we need to get back to the hotel." Ravit acceded but, ever since, "I've been having these thoughts that I missed out on something by not going into the synagogue and that I need to go back there." Four members entered the playing space. The first expressed the feeling of missing out by not having entered the synagogue: "why didn't I insist? There is a piece of me missing." The second member expressed the feeling of uncanny longing for the abandoned synagogue: "it felt like there was something mystical about it. Something that's still drawing me there. As if I know this place from another life." The third member expressed anger toward Ravit's impatient husband and children: "why are they always so stubborn about having things their way!" And the fourth member expressed a sense of acceptance mixed with sadness: "I understand that we had to move on and that there's nothing you can do, sometimes you need to make concessions for your family, but I wish it didn't have to be that way." Placing these four voices side by side gives them equal weight in the teller's explicit emotional experience and allows voices that are often silenced to be on an equal footing with voices that are usually more prominent in one's experience. In response, Ravit recalled her prolonged experience of growing up as an older sister to two twin brothers, whose needs constantly forced Ravit to make concessions. She spoke about her experience of accepting and acknowledging the need to make concessions as well as feeling angry and sad about the experiences she had to give up.

Content structuring

This form of structuring is done by dividing the contents of the story and its interpretations and assigning each a different location. As mentioned, in the "arrowhead" pattern, the front part usually represents the more conscious aspects, while the two rear parts usually represent less conscious aspects which, as such, are more open to the interpretation of the playing members. Various psychotherapeutic theories can also be applied in this manner. For example, the Freudian theory of the psychic apparatus can be grafted onto this pattern by positioning the ego in front of the playing space, while placing the id and the super-ego in the back; in a relational context, conscious possible self-states can be positioned downstage, while less conscious self-states are relegated upstage, to the back of the playing space.

This is illustrated through the story shared by Milly, a 35-year-old woman, who told the group that, about a month ago, her husband received his PhD degree with honors. She talked about wanting to throw a surprise party with friends and family to celebrate this event, but never being able to find the right time for the party itself or for all the necessary arrangements.

This week is all busy and so is next week, with classes and other things the children have to attend, and I can already see the weeks just passing by and it's not happening and it's been a month now and I simply can't see it happening and I'm disappointed in myself. I also find it so strange, because it's usually very easy for me to make these things happen.

For the theatrical response, the members chose the "arrowhead" pattern. One member stood at the front of the playing space and explained, very reasonably, that the schedule was jam packed with so many things with the kids that it was hard to find a good time to throw a party, "maybe in summer, when things cool down... but in summer everything is so hectic because the kids are home... so next year..." The second member stood behind them and to their right and voiced Milly's moral agony: "what kind of wife am I, if I'm not thrilled that my husband is doing so well, if I can't put something together to celebrate his success. How hard is it to throw a party?" A third member stood behind her and to her left, and voiced Milly's feelings of envy and anger toward her husband:

he went off to fulfill himself in academia and I got stuck with the kids and all their classes. I'm supposed to throw *him* a party... He should throw *me* a party... if things were the other way around, I would have gotten real far, but someone had to stay home while he travelled to all those important conferences of his.

In response to this theatrical response, Milly smiled bashfully and said: "there were some meaningful parts that you showed on stage, even though I didn't tell you about them." She talked about her desire to go back to school and her feeling that there is never time for that. She talked about how agonizing it is for her to take time to do the things she is interested in – "I feel like it's always at the children's expense" – and about envying her husband for allowing himself to move ahead in life. Later on, the group began discussing the way in which feelings of envy are delegitimized, even though they entail significant desires and wishes. This vignette shows that dividing the story into distinct voices, in a manner that is also grounded in a particular theoretical perspective, allows a deeper exploration of the story's hidden voices and the teller's experience.

Chronological structuring

This form of structuring involves dividing the narrative into beginning, middle and end, presenting a focused theatrical representation of each part and then reintegrating all three parts into a single flow. Three members enter the playing space and each, in turn, presents a theatrical representation, with voice and movement, of a certain part of the story: one will present a motif from the beginning of the story, another a motif from the middle of the story and the third a motif from the end of the story. By showing all three motifs in the playing space and linking them through movement, the theatrical response facilitates the integration of the various components. Another kind of chronological structuring can be achieved through the presentation of different life periods – childhood, youth, adulthood and old age. Chronological reintegration is often done by moving between the different theatrical representations positioned around the playing space, in an attempt to reorganize the various aspects of the story. For example, consider the story of 77-year-old Rachel, who shared a story about her childhood in Russia, where she grew up with a physically abusive mother. When she immigrated to Israel, she got married and had children of her own and managed to raise a family that was free of violence. Later on, she started working as a custodian at a boarding school and did very well at her job, teaching the children and caring for their needs. The group created a dramatic image that featured three characters – the little girl, the mother and the teacher-caretaker – each of whom delivered her own monologue. The figure of the teller as a little girl came in the playing space first: she lay bundled up in a corner, clasping a cloth doll in her arms and said, "Sometimes, at night, I dream about a different family, a family that one is happy to come home to, where mom hugs me at night when I cry." Then the figure of the teller as a mother came in the playing space, walked up to the little girl, caressed her cheek and then took her cloth and turned it into a kind of child-figure. She gazed at it with warmth and tenderness and said, "my boy, I'm so glad that I have you." Then, the figure of the teller as custodian came into the playing space, turned to the members sitting in the audience as if they were the children at the boarding school and said, "we don't get to choose the family we are born into, but we can choose what we do about it, we can choose the life we build for ourselves." Finally, custodian-Rachel turned to girl-Rachel and said,

> look at how much you've grown in life, how you've managed to overcome everything you had been through and build a different life for yourself and your children. The three playing members were very moved throughout the theatrical response and, when it reached its end, they embraced. In response, Rachel said, "there was so much love on stage. Exactly the kind of love I lacked as a child."

This vignette shows how chronological structuring can serve to emphasize the elements of continuity, growth and reparation in the teller's life.

Partially planned theatrical response

As the therapeutic process progresses, the group's need for structuring de-creases. One can gradually shift from using pre-determined patterns as a container to more open improvisation, which does not conform to any pre-made pattern, in which the whole group can work on the story shared by one member. In the initial stages of the transition to improvising without a pre-determined pattern, the group still has a certain need for structuring and it is advised to work within the framework of a partially planned improvisation.

In this form of structuring, the group is divided into several small sub-groups, each of which functions as a group of playing members who re-act to the story with their own theatrical response. All sub-groups reflect a single story, which is told to the entire group. The sub-groups are given a short amount of time to prepare a rough outline of their theatrical response and then each sub-group presents its piece. This method allows all group members to work and to experiment with performing and encountering the story. In addition, such a variety of theatrical responses offers multiple perspectives on the story. The role of the conductor at this stage is to guide the sub-groups through the different stages of planning their theatrical piece. For example, they may ask members to contemplate the main theme of the story and the ways in which it can be translated into dramatic language, the specification of the external characters and inner voices, the choice of music and use of cloths as well as at which point in the story the theatrical response should begin and end.

In a brief and limited amount of time, the members plan a synopsis of the theatrical response. However, before the sub-groups begin planning, the conductor may ask the teller a series of questions that will help the other members be better attuned to the teller's experience as well as give a certain measure of control over their story back to them. The teller is also asked to choose which member will play their character in each sub-group, as well as to discuss themselves as a character – "why don't you tell us about [tell-er's name] in this story?" (the use of the third person is designed to create greater distance for the teller). For example, a teller who shares a childhood story about his grandmother's house is asked: "please tell us about Nir, the boy who is visiting his grandmother." Next, the other members are invited to ask the teller informative questions about their story. It is important not to overwhelm the teller with questions and to choose questions that will indeed help the members create their theatrical response. In most cases, questions about the story are avoided so as not to lead the members to cognitive, concrete and emotionally distanced thinking about the story. The aim is to keep the teller in the same emotional mood that resulted from their spontaneously telling of their story. Finally, the teller is asked to pick a name for their story.

After the teller has provided all the necessary information, the members are given a short time to plan and then perform their theatrical response. It is important to keep the planning phase short and focused. The members can be instructed to avoid any attempt at a psychological analysis of the teller and the story and to focus rather on dramatic decisions, such as the order of events, the key images and so on. Once the theatrical response is concluded, the members remain in the playing space and look at the teller. This look entails a symbolic act of returning the story to the teller and turning the emotional attention to them and their response to the improvisation.

There are three levels of structuring for the partially planned theatrical response. The first involves the definition, specification and pre-selection of all the story's characters and the members who will play them; the second involves the specification only of the character of the teller and the pre-selection of the member who will play them; the third involves no pre-selection of any story's character or member. At this level of structuring, each member spontaneously chooses which character they want to play as well as how to play it. A detailed example of a partially planned theatrical response can be found in Chapter 10.

Open theatrical improvisation

This is the most open type of improvisation in Psychotherapeutic Playback Theater. It bears the most similarity to the free-association technique of psychoanalysis as it invited members to free-associate to the story in various ways. The playing members can choose when to enter the playing space, where they position themselves, the manner in which they reflect the story and react to the other members, which dramatic role to play, how the various elements will be integrated, the musical accompaniment, etc.

Group members sit in a semi-circle facing the playing space. One member shares their story while the group listens. Once the story is over, the conductor and the other members may ask the teller questions, as depicted above. Once again, it is stressed that it is better to ask fewer questions – or even none at all. Next, the members enter the playing space and present a free improvisation in response to the story. This theatrical response may entail various elements, from a theatrical reflection to images and metaphors, texts, songs and music that are associatively related to the story; the manifold perspectives of the characters and objects mentioned in the story; emotions, dreams and desires; any artistic material that resonates the story in the eyes of the playing members. Members enter and exit the playing space. Each time they enter the playing space, a member can express their association to the story either by themselves or by directing and engaging other group members. Members may freely enter and leave the playing space and may combine their associations, have them interact with each other through dialogue, duplication or resonance, or present them side by side. This way of working, in which the playing space is always open, facilitates a flow of free associations that are linked to the psychic material expressed in the story as well as the web of relationships that has been established between the group members.

In Psychotherapeutic Playback Theater, open improvisation invites considerable richness into the process and the resulting theatrical piece. The individual tells their story and, in response, many different things emerge in the playing space. In many cases, the members feel the need to express a great number of theatrical associations following their encounter with the story. However, one must keep in mind that an excessive variety of dramatic events may be overwhelming and lead to under-structuring and therefore also bring about under-containment and a failure to address many of the story's ideas.

Note that it is important to maintain the aesthetic and the narrative containers in open improvisations as well, though in a "slacker" manner. As far as the *aesthetic container* is concerned, the composition or mise-en-scène of the various members throughout the various parts of the playing space (downstage, upstage, center stage, left and right) is very important. As mentioned, the explicit elements of the story will often be presented downstage, while the implicit parts, the urges and the inner voices, will be presented upstage. These notions correspond with Bromberg's (1993) conceptualization of *multiple self-states,* which is highly useful in contemplating the formal aesthetics of the open improvisation and even the structure and form of pre-determined patterns and the partially planned theatrical response. Bromberg (ibid.) likens the psyche to a stage, in which there is a figure-ground relation between downstage and upstage. Potential self-states that are closer to the front of the stage are experienced as a more dominant part of one's conscious sense of self (figure), while potential self-states that are more upstage or on the sides of the stage are experienced as less dominant in one's conscious sense of self. These self-states affect one's emotional experience by creating a less conscious context (ground) in which the figure is perceived. This context affects one in an implicit, unconscious and peripheral manner, but its impact on one's experience and one's perception of the figure is crucial.

The presence of the aesthetic container can be augmented by turning the attention of the members to the dramatic composition or mise-en-scène. It is important to do so in a way that offers further inspiration to work openly and associatively, rather than as strict, evaluative and judgmental feedback, which may hinder the associative richness of the members. In this context, one should remember that, like any other container, the aesthetic container can also lead to stifling and limiting "over-containment" and that it, too, should occasionally be tempered and even breached throughout the process. For this purpose, members can practice creating spontaneous playing space compositions that are unprompted by stories (the structuring of playing space compositions based on a variety of stories is demonstrated in Chapter 6). In addition, one can turn the attention of the members to the compositions that emerge spontaneously in open theatrical improvisations or discuss these and their psychic significance when one is verbally recapitulating the sequence of story or a series of stories.

As far as the *narrative container* is concerned, one can focus on the narrative structure that emerges spontaneously in the improvisation or turn the members' attention to potential narrative structures that may help them time their entrances into the playing space within the general sequence. It is important that this indication, too, is presented as a suggestion rather than formulated as a strict set of rules that might limit creative and associative freedom. Certain classic narrative structures, which are grounded in Greek theater, were mentioned in Chapter 2 on theatrical mirroring.

We will now present an additional narrative structure, which is highly useful in inspiring open theatrical improvisations. It draws on the classic narrative structure, as presented in Aristotle's *Poetics*, while also integrating certain structural notions from the realm of object-relations and from Melanie Klein's theory of the two positions (1975).

a   *Expressing the Conscious Emotional Atmosphere* – The teller should be able to recognize themselves emotionally and feel emotionally seen from the very outset of the theatrical response. This expression corresponds to the experience that accompanies the object-relations system, which Klein describes as "the emotional atmosphere surrounding the object-relation system" (1975). This aspect is often present in the teller's conscious experience, sometimes unaccountably so. The expression of the conscious emotional feeling serves as a kind of emotional bridge connecting the teller and the theatrical response and the other members.

b   *Elaborating Inner World Expressions* – Images, associations, internalized objects and object-relations, various potential self-states, archetypes, etc., form the greater share of the theatrical response. This part explores the members' associations to the inner world manifest in the story, resulting in the potential elaboration of different possible elements and points of view of the inner world.

c   *The Anxiety which Lies in the Story* – More often than not, the stories introduced on the playing space of Psychotherapeutic Playback Theater implicitly entail unconscious anxieties, which prominently inform the teller's unconscious conduct. The exploration of the inner world often exposes and expresses these anxieties as part of the theatrical response.

d   *Intervention* – This part corresponds to Klein's (1975) notion of *the wish for reparation*, Moreno's (1961) notion of *surplus reality* and Landy's (1993) notion of *the guide*. At this stage, the members offer interventions which alter the narrative by heightening weak or silenced voices, integrating split-off parts, introducing new perspectives on the story, etc. During the intervention stage, it is important to consider the extent of the gap between the proposed interventions and the external and internal reality presented by the teller, in order to try and limit instances of *manic reparation*, which denies certain parts of this reality and eventually leads to a sense of alienation and loneliness (Klein, 1975). For example, if a member were to tell a story about how painful it was to lose her father and about all the things she never got to tell him, the theatrical response would do well to present the pain and the sense of missing out, which are explicitly mentioned in the story. While a meeting of father and daughter or the conversation that never took place can also be proposed in the theatrical response, these should not be presented without expressing the absence and its concomitant sense of loss.

e   *Integration* – The recapitulation and integration of the various parts mentioned thus far, especially the anxiety and the intervention. This part leads to the concluding image of the theatrical response, which seeks to piece together the different parts and also contains a prospect of the future.

The following vignette describes a process that follows this narrative structure. Maya, a 45-year-old woman, described having difficulties dealing with the loss of her mother, who passed away a year before. Maya depicted saying goodbye to her mother after a protracted illness as well as her everyday life since then and her immense feelings of longing and lack at the absence of their conversations and family dinners. Maya shared with the group how badly she wanted to seek her mother's advice, how terribly lonely she felt and how great the void was. The conductor invited the group to create an open theatrical improvisation, in which each member can enter the group stage whenever they wish and freely present any dramatic association in response to the story. The theatrical response began with a song about a mother-daughter relationship, a song that had an elegiac and sentimental emotional quality – the same as Maya's story. Then, two playing members took the playing space and presented a shared dance: the two women held two differently colored cloths, passing them from one to the other until they finally became tied together, forming a kind of umbilical cord that connected the two women. Then, another member came up and gave a monologue that manifested a feeling of anger at the loss and absence, anger toward the universe, toward the mother, toward the sense of having been abandoned and toward the loneliness one was left to endure. Another member came up to face him and introduced the guilt of forgetting. Next, a playing member came into the playing space holding a bowl filled with water. He tried to keep the water from spilling over, but some inevitably spilled on the floor at every step. Each time, he stopped in a panic, looking at the water that had been irretrievably spilled. After a few steps, he started a monologue about how hard it is to hold on to a memory: "you're constantly with me, I try to remember you always, but sometimes I just can't." Finally, a group of playing members entered the playing space and presented a memory of a Friday night dinner: gathered for a holiday feast around a table, covered with a colorful cloth in lieu of a tablecloth, they sang a song together. They chose a traditional Jewish song – "how good and how pleasant it is for brothers and sisters to dwell together in unity" – that emphasized the strong family values that the mother had held for the entire family, values that are present in Maya's life today, that she has been upholding for her own family and her own children.

Beginning the theatrical response with a song represents the first stage of the narrative container by reflecting the story's *explicit emotional quality*. This helps the teller recognize their emotional experience and makes them feel validated and seen. This initial stage allows the teller to be more available and receptive toward the more interpretative and self-reflective parts, later in the theatrical response. Next, we see the parts in which the group presents images that offer various potential interpretations of *the teller's inner world*: the image of the shared dance around the umbilical cord, representing her relationship with her mother, as well as images of the inner voices expressing anger and loneliness, etc. This part of the theatrical response thereby illustrates the second stage of the proposed structure for a narrative container. This part then evolves into the third stage of the structure, through the image of the gradually emptying bowl of water and the expression of helplessness in the face of one's diminishing memories. These manifest the *anxiety* which is at the root of the experience of loss – the anxiety of losing any representation of or connection to the internal object corresponding to the person one has lost. The memory of the family dinner serves as an *intervention* and thus represents the fourth stage of the structure. It functions as a counterweight for the anxiety by indicating the significance of the memory and its continuity despite the loss. The simultaneous presence of anxiety and reparation on a single playing space represents the fifth stage of the narrative container, because it allows for the *integration* of the terror of emptiness and the experience of remembrance and continuity.

In Psychotherapeutic Playback Theater, open improvisation encourages the flow of associations between members and offers a formal expression of the events and resonances. It creates flexible and spontaneous aesthetic containers for the personal and group processes, which are manifest in unpremeditated modes of formal organization in the playing space. There is considerable overlap between these forms and the group's levels of discourse (Schlapobersky, 2016) – monologues, synchronized monologues, dialogues and discourse. *Monologues* feature members entering the playing space one after the other, sometimes even occupying the very same spot or area, to express their dramatic associations in a sequence of solo performances. This organization involves no dialogue between simultaneous associations on the dramatic level, but rather an associative sequence that is presented diachronically. In the theatrical response, the spontaneous structuring of *synchronized monologues* has two members coming up into the playing space and presenting their dramatic associations simultaneously. While this structure involves no explicit dialogue between the members occupying the playing space, it does create a certain synchronicity by virtue of their "simultaneity." This synchronicity creates an aesthetic container which facilitates the linking of associations in preparation for the emergence of new thinking. These synchronized monologues may evolve into a *dialogue* – two members are simultaneously present in the playing space and are fueled by each other's associations. Sometimes, the playing space may see the emergence of the *discourse* as a formal container, with several members acting simultaneously and fueled by one another's associations. The levels of dramatic discourse and the formal-aesthetic container created by the members express and inform the group process. These levels allow one to identify both those contents around which there is an increase in group cohesion and those which diminish cohesion, but nevertheless serve as an opportunity, as a new beta-element which may lead to the tempering of the old container and the creation of a new one.

Levels of structuring during the teller's response and the post-response sharing circle

Once the theatrical response is over, the group's attention returns to the teller, who may now respond to what they have seen. At higher levels of structuring, the conductor may ask the teller about those parts of the theatrical response that are closer or more distant in relation to their experience. The conductor may ask the teller if they would like to change anything about the theatrical response – to heighten, specify or altogether eliminate a certain voice or detail, to lead the theatrical response down a certain path, to focus on certain contents, etc. At lower levels of structuring, the conductor will address the teller and ask them to keep resonating the associations that surfaced in the playing space by providing their own associations to them. It should be noted that, in many cases, the teller is left speechless after the theatrical response. In such cases, one should consider transitioning into a *sharing circle* that would help them find words for what they are feeling or trying to encourage them to say a few words or some short sentences. Both the sharing circle and the handful of words spoken by the teller serve as a container for their experiences after watching the theatrical response. Even when the teller says nothing, however, it is very important to return the attention to them once the theatrical response is over; this act actually returns the story to their possession after it was borrowed from them in order to facilitate the group's associations.

After both the theatrical response and the teller's response are concluded, the conductor invites everyone to share verbally the ways in which the story resonates in their own lives. It is important for the sharing circle to focus on the way this emotional experience resonates in the lives of the other members, rather than on any advice or interpretation they might offer. The sharing circle often creates a powerful experience of intimacy and acceptance for the teller. It recapitulates the dramatic reflection in words, thus granting it the form of a more solid and clear container. It also serves to call everyone back from the realm of primary, associative and surreal thinking, which was manifest in the theatrical response, to the domain of real-life stories and secondary thinking. The sharing circle helps members own and mark those parts of their inner world that resonate with the teller's inner world. This creates the experience of being intimate-while-separate, which involves an *exchange* of psychic material, while limiting the experience of being intimate-while-blended, which involves *merger* and is more characteristic of the theatrical response. After the sharing circle is over, the group once again returns to the teller for a brief and concluding response. As mentioned, this aims to give them back their ownership of that part of the session that was created in response to their story and explored their psychic contents and to resume the exchange of psychic material with a greater degree of separateness.

In conclusion, this chapter depicted the possibilities of the therapeutic process as a process that structures aesthetic and narrative containers for arising psychic material. The different forms of structuring range from more to less structured processes along the spectrum. The aim is to enable a flexible and dynamic container which is adapted to the group process and which invites the introduction of new psychic material to the group within a developmental and creative process. This therapeutic function embodies the dramatic-aesthetic qualities that are at the very core of the Psychotherapeutic Playback Theater process and thus forms a key axis of the therapeutic process.

Chapter 8

Theatrical forms in Psychotherapeutic Playback Theater[1]

Ronen Kowalsky, Nir Raz, Shoshi Keisari

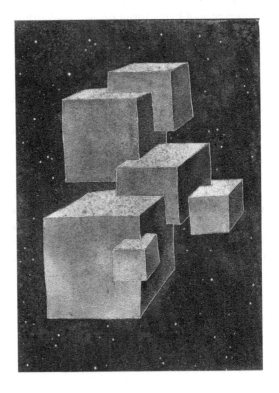

Figure 8.1

The various stages of the creative process serve as a space in which group dynamics unfold. This process creates a shared experience and a mutual engagement between group members: starting with the introduction of the personal story that emerges in group space, through the encounter between the story and the members, the improvisation and the resulting theatrical

DOI: 10.4324/9781003167822-9

response, to giving the story back to the teller and the sharing circle. This chapter focuses on a key aspect of this process – the use of structuring through theatrical forms as a means of promoting developmental tasks within the group process. In this chapter, we will introduce typical playback theatrical forms and their connection to group stages in line with the model presented by MacKenzie and Livesley (1983).

Theatrical forms are predefined structures that provide an aesthetic framework and an enveloping container for theatrical response. They are known and familiar to the group members and the conductor. Members may use this to cast the contents of the story into a theatrical response that has a recognizable structure. These forms were developed by the originator of Playback Theater, Jonathan Fox (Rowe, 2007), and are also known as "short forms." In cases where members have little experience in acting in general or Playback Theater in particular, these forms (such as *chorus, duet* and *sculpture;* a detailed description of these forms will be given later in this chapter) can help in developing their acting and improvisation skills by offering a clear definition of the kind of response required as well as the role each member should play. It is important to mention that improvisation processes, which are grounded in working within a theatrical form, represent a high level of structuring (see level of structuring axis in the previous chapter).

The theatrical form acts as a container for psychic material and expresses contents that are adapted to the various stages of the group. Selected in response to the personal story, the theatrical form enables the exploration of the group process as well as the self, in its encounter with the others in the group. The person sees themselves or parts of themselves reflected back to them through the others in the group (Foulkes, 1964). In this sense, the theatrical form is a manifestation of different kinds of mirroring processes. The choice of a particular theatrical form may push group processes forward by coping with various developmental tasks. Thus, this choice serves the conductor as an instrument for intervention in the group process, in a manner that supports its progression.

Theatrical forms express concrete aspects of the story alongside thoughts, emotions and inner voices, the perspectives of additional characters, movement, music and imagery. The process of theatrical response is comprised of dividing the story into its various elements, creating a theatrical representation of each element and reconstructing the story through the integration of all the elements within a pre-existing theatrical form. On a psychic level, the deconstruction of the plot and its ensuing reconstruction by means of structured forms enable the elucidation and reorganization of the emotional world expressed in the story. This process allows the conductor and the group to restructure the personal and group stories. The act of deconstructing and reconstructing the myriad voices emerging from the story and arranging them into a pre-determined aesthetic theatrical form transforms the material and creates a container for the contents of the story. The story expands and takes on new dimensions, revealing new points of view. The teller is acknowledged for their story and learns to acknowledge its value.

Theatrical forms are integrated into group work in the following manner: members listen to the story one of them shares. As mentioned in previous chapters, they are initially requested to relate to the feelings this story evokes in them, through its encounter with their inner world, their life experience and similar experiences they have had either in the group or outside of it. Next, the explicit and implicit elements of the story are presented through theatrical representation and are integrated via a theatrical form chosen by the conductor or the members.

The personal story introduced into the group leads to the creation of a collective experience; it is encountered by others and becomes part of a shared group experience. The theatrical forms help the therapist highlight or selectively initiate certain behaviors that are appropriate to the developmental stage of the group. As described by Anthony and Foulkes (1965), the most important role of the conductor is to help the group pool and become familiar with its resources. Structured theatrical forms facilitate exploration of and more profound engagement with the developmental tasks relevant to each stage. While these forms are pre-determined, they can also be used modularly, like toy blocks. Different forms can be created to address emerging needs and heighten inner voices in accordance with the group process and its developmental stage. The conductor can thereby help the group tackle its developmental tasks and push forward.

In fact, theatrical forms constitute active therapeutic interventions through theatrical action. For example, when the conductor notices a lack in the teller's inner world, they can be offered a way of coping with this lack through the theatrical mean. Theatrical forms allow one to focus, to heighten an inner voice, to reorganize narratives and relationships, to integrate split-off internal voices and more. Finally, theatrical forms serve to connect group members to a broader social context, which also makes room for the group unconscious. Thus, the material arising through theatrical response provides a fertile ground for initiating changes in the group. As noted by Beck (1981), the fabric of the developing social system and individual events creates a significant momentum for change. Theatrical response renders group forces – and sometimes even the unconscious parts subsisting in group space – tangibly present, thereby allowing the group, led by the conductor, to observe and engage these directly.

Stages of group development according to MacKenzie

The majority of theories concerning groups view the group process as unfolding in stages (e.g., Bion, 1961; MacKenzie and Livesley, 1983; Tuckman,

1965; Yalom and Leszcz, 2005). Each developmental stage or phase undergone by the group involves its own distinct issues and conflicts, which require different coping methods. This section focuses on theatrical forms and their relation to the developmental model for brief group therapy proposed by MacKenzie and Livesley (1983), in order to describe the therapeutic processes that take place in Psychotherapeutic Playback Theater groups through work with such forms.

MacKenzie (1990) describes three independent dimensions for assessing groups: *engagement*, *avoidance* and *conflict*. The theatrical representations emerging in the group process of Psychotherapeutic Playback Theater manifest these three dimensions. Each particular theatrical form manifests these different dimensions in varying ratios, in accordance with the needs arising from the process. Playback Theater offers a tangible stage, on which group processes and the issues emerging from each developmental stage are played out.

The developmental model put forward by MacKenzie and Livesley (1983) serves as an overarching theory that lists six phases of development in time-limited groups: *(1) Engagement*; *(2) Differentiation*; *(3) Individuation*; *(4) Intimacy*; *(5) Mutuality* and *(6) Termination*. Group dynamics are expressed at each stage of the process as well as during the theatrical improvisation performed in response to the teller's personal story. The manner in which the theatrical response unfolds also serves as a space in which group dynamics expresses itself and the conductor may offer interventions. Therefore, the theatrical forms chosen by the conductor or the group may, in and of themselves, serve as a space for exploring the group process, in accordance with the group's present developmental stage.

Theatrical forms according to Mackenzie's stages of group development

In this section, we will elaborate on typical theatrical forms, demonstrating their structure, their therapeutic rationale and their connection to group stages in line with the model presented by MacKenzie and Livesley (1983). While the stories emerging in the group are very diverse, the group's attitude toward the story corresponds to its attitude toward the present developmental stage. Finding the appropriate theatrical form for the group's present stage will be the best way to serve the story because, in many cases, both the personal story and the way in which the group uses it to work are a reflection of the group process.

The role of the conductor is to call forth theatrical forms that could serve as a space of exploration and experience for the members and the material the group gives rise to, in accordance with its developmental stage. In this chapter, we will present five common theatrical forms: *chorus, duet, cross, shared dance* and *sculpture*.

Chorus

This pattern is appropriate for the first stage of the model – that of *engagement*. At this stage, the wish is to form a group, to blur one's individuality in favor of collectivity and of those aspects that are shared by all group members. The chorus form finds shared elements and acts as an "emotional and instinctual amplifier," through shared voice and movement work. This form highlights the relinquishment of individual uniqueness in favor of collectivity and structures group cohesion and uniformity through the element of synchronization. In the chorus, synchronization is realized as a form of coordinated behavior, in which the behavior patterns of distinct people become a single, coordinated and unified pattern (Bernieri & Rosenthal, 1991).

This form is inspired by the Greek chorus, which was part of the structure of Greek tragedy. The play took place at the center of the stage, while at the side of the stage was the chorus, whose role was to shed light on various points of the story, emphasize certain parts in it and express its hidden and implicit elements (Walcot, 1976). The chorus makes use of such artistic devices as singing, movement and imagery. It connects the different parts of the plot while also driving it forward, by reporting battles or historical events that had taken place but were not actually shown in the playing space. Some of the other roles of the Greek chorus included coming in during moments of peak tension in the plot and alleviating it, encouraging the audience to think and take a stand, and stating the moral of the play.

Structure

Three or four members stand in a semi-circle, so that they are able to see one another. They stand shoulder to shoulder, in close contact so as to form a single entity. They listen to the story told by another member, picking up on emotional keywords or words that represent the story's main themes. It is best to use only one or two words, rather than long sentences, in order to maintain the form's rhythm and technique.

The prime goal of the chorus is to achieve unity and synchronization. The members of the chorus begin by taking three breaths together, symbolizing that "we are one." After these breaths, one member says a word or two from the story, adding a movement that expresses the emotional experience this word evokes. Once the first word has been said, the other members count to two in their heads and then everyone utters the word together, as a coordinated chorus. In this manner, they repeat the word three times and then move on to a new word that expresses another element from the story. Words are not spoken according to the order in which the story unfolded but emerge in a jumbled fashion – much like inner voices, thoughts and feelings.

The psychic notion represented by the chorus is that of an emotional amplifier. The amplification stems from the shared repetition of key elements from the story. The chorus adds various elements which are joined together to form one complete and amplified picture. The chorus also reinforces the connection between members by drawing on synchronization and the integration of different voices.

Duet

This form corresponds to the second stage of the developmental model, that of *differentiation*, which involves the need of the members to emphasize that they are different and separate. During this stage, there is more room for divergence and there is an emerging sense of "not being like everyone else." This stage is characterized by conflicts that highlight the boundaries and differences between group members. The duet form allows two distinct voices to be heard in a single space, while neither of them listens to the other and each is preoccupied with their own position. The conductor can invite stories about conflicts and members will often share stories that reflect the group process even without being directly asked to do so.

Structure

One of the group members shares a story that features distinct, contrasting voices; for example, a conversation between a mother and her son. In this technique, two members stand in the playing space facing the audience, about two feet apart. One member plays the teller, while the other member plays the role of the mother. The member playing the teller starts sharing his view of what had happened with the audience. At some point, the other member, the one playing the mother, interrupts the first member and tells the audience what happened from their perspective. They continue until they are interrupted by the first member and the two continue to shift the focus between them until the conductor calls out "freeze" or until they have finished telling their stories.

This form allows two opposing voices to inhabit the same space side by side. Each of them recounts their own perspective, in the belief that they are telling the truth. Another aspect of this form is the mobilization of the audience in support of a certain viewpoint, as each character is trying to convince the audience that they are right while the other is wrong. Thus, the duet form emphasizes both what one is projecting onto the other and what one believes the other is thinking about them.

Cross

This form corresponds to the third stage of the developmental model – *individuation*. At this stage, each member's individual personality is expressed in the group, giving rise to issues such as how can individuals form a group and how to make space for distinct voices within the group without erasing the individual. This form calls for an exploration of additional parts of the self, alongside an active interpersonal challenge within a supportive environment, as part of the individuation stage. For more details on this theatrical form and other forms that represent conflicts and contradictions, see Chapter 4.

Structure

After one of the members has shared a story that entails a conflict or opposing emotions, two members stand at the two ends of the playing space, very far apart, facing the audience. In the first few beats of this form, it is important for them to avoid making eye contact with one another. Each member picks a clear and well-defined side of the conflict. The first member gives a brief monologue, comprising two to three sentences, and takes a single step sideways, toward the center of the playing space. In turn, the other member gives a brief monologue advocating the opposite position and takes a step toward the center. In this manner, the two members continue to move toward the center, while trying to win the audience to their perspective. At some point, the two members meet at the center of the playing space. This is a crucial stage, in which the two voices meet each other for the first time: the two members see one another, look at each other and take in their difference. They exchange materials. At this point, while still facing and looking at each other, they move in a semi-circle and assume each other's position as well as the other's viewpoint. Then, they begin stepping outward, while trying to convince the audience of their newfound truth – which is the opposite of the position they started with. This form illustrates the possibility for two sides to co-exist in the same space, even when each of them holds a different truth. They may even enrich each other and exchange psychic materials.

Shared dance

This form matches the fourth and fifth stages of the developmental model – those of *intimacy* and *mutuality* – offering a tangible illustration of them. At these stages, one feels drawn precisely to someone who is different from them and intimacy is grounded in the acknowledgment of difference. This form allows us to raise questions such as how one can expand one's limits through the other. Difference serves as a potential for self-expansion and is experienced as less of a threat.

Structure

A group member shares a story to which everyone listens. While music corresponding to the emotional mood of the story is playing in the background, three members enter the playing space. Initially, each member offers a movement phrase that expresses a different part of the story. After a short while, they move to the second part of the form, in which they form a kind of movement dialogue, a kind of dance through which they explore the movements already established. The intimacy created in this dance stems from the playing members "almost touching" one another: they move together within the various movements, finding different types of connections. The third part of the form does involve touch, as the three members become a single body, moving in unison. The aim of this form is to show how difference can invite dialogue and intimacy and lead to a freely chosen connection, as well as how dialogue creates a new movement that stems from the linking of different movements.

"Past, present, future" sculpture

This form corresponds to the sixth stage of the developmental model – *termination* – which entails recapitulation and the working through of separation processes. The past-present-future sculpture form symbolizes the development of the individual, from previous life stages, through the "here and now," to a position of looking toward the future. This form allows the conductor and the group to observe the co-existence of different aspects of the self, which manifest development. From this vantage point, the group accepts personal exploration as a legitimate and even important part of group development.

Structure

Group members listen to the story one of them has chosen to tell. After the teller presents their story, the conductor interviews them, trying to get answers to two key questions: (1) How does this story relate to the past? (2) How do they imagine this story developing in the future?

Three members perform the form, after deciding in advance which of them will play past, present and future. Members stand at the back of the playing space. Each of them, in turn, performs a short monologue, adding a movement that captures the relevant aspect of the story. The first member presents a movement and a monologue that symbolize the past. After they are done, they create a sculpture that captures the emotional state of the chosen monologue. The second member offers a movement and a monologue symbolizing the present and, while doing so, directly or indirectly relates to the sculpture of the past that is already in the playing space. After they finish, they create a sculpture that is added and joined to the sculpture made by the first member. The third member presents the future aspect of the story through their movement and monologue and then creates a sculpture. The third member should take into account that, because they are symbolizing the continuation of the story, their monologue should include a message of hope, reference to significant milestones, expectation and open-ness. Once they are done, they join the shared sculpture and all three members maintain a brief freeze.

The final part of the form involves the sculpture reawakening and coming back to life. The three parts come to life, each of them intently focused on their own monologue, as if to say: "my part is the most meaningful part of the story." After some 30 seconds, they create a new shared sculpture and maintain it for a ten-second freeze, in order for the teller and the audience to take in the entire sculpture, which embodies this new development. Once the theatrical response is finished, the group engages in a sharing circle that allows members to express stories and feelings that the emerging story and the theatrical response evoked in them, as well as feelings, emotions and thoughts arising from the process as a whole.

Suggested interventions through theatrical forms

In this section, we will present suggested interventions using theatrical forms in accordance with the group's developmental stage. It should be noted that, just as the stages of group development are not entirely distinct and the group is often engaged in developmental tasks belonging to earlier stages, theatrical forms are also not as clear-cut. The suggested interventions draw on the characteristics of the theatrical pattern, the type of relations it represents and the present stage of the group. However, it goes without saying that one can also use different forms or utilize the suggested forms at a different point in the group process, in line with the considerations of the conductor and the needs of the group. For example, the conflict (Cross) form may also serve the group during the mutuality stage, if the group needs to resort to it. At any stage, forms can be remolded to fit the needs arising from the story and the group process.

Moreover, there are many more common and well-known theatrical forms that are used in Playback Theater and in Psychotherapeutic Playback Theater. The conductors and the members (re)create them every time, in relation to new needs. They can be altered to address the need arising from the story and the group process.

Therefore, this section will discuss the possibilities available to the conductor in selecting theatrical forms as a means for promoting group processes, as illustrated by three random sessions – used here as typical examples – from Psychotherapeutic Playback Theater groups for adults. The process entails 24 weekly sessions, each three hours long. The following events are inspired by actual groups, but have been altered to remove any identifying details.

In the group's second session, Jason told the other members about a job he is about to start at a new workplace. He has been waiting for such a career change for a long time and now, as its growing closer, he is experiencing considerable anxiety and fear of failure. The theatrical form chosen by the conductor to reflect the voices arising from this story was the *chorus*. The aim was to give these voices back and highlight the extent to which other members relate to this story. Each member was asked to echo a single phrase that expresses their connection to the story. One member chose to echo the phrase "change"; another chose "I'm so afraid"; the third chose "what if I don't make it..."; and the fourth said "I've waited, I want this." The members amplified these voices and repeated them, in sync, in accordance with the chorus form.

The chorus form made it possible to emphasize the shared universal experience of the members, an experience they all acknowledged, thus promoting mutual engagement. The teller felt that his story and the different voices he introduced were acknowledged and validated. Alongside this, the story and theatrical response it inspired reflected the group process and the position of the members – *the engagement stage*. At this stage, feelings of expectation and desire surrounding the beginning of the process arise alongside an inevitable sense of anxiety. The intervention through the chorus form, which highlights the similarity between members, reinforced the experience of universality and thus helped the group tackle its developmental task.

In the group's seventh session, Claudia shared a story about a conflict between her and her life partner. She described a situation they experienced several months earlier, in an old house they were renovating. She was the one who chose that house, while her partner would have preferred to move into a comfortable new apartment. About two months after they moved in, after the house had been thoroughly renovated, the roots of a nearby old tree broke into the pipes, causing a sewage overflow in their new house. Faced with this major mishap, the couple felt that their safe place – their home – was undermined, giving rise to doubts about the shared decisions they had made as well as feelings of insecurity and helplessness. This conflict highlighted their choices in the face of reality and the role each of them played in the decision-making process.

During that time, in terms of the group process, the group was in the *differentiation* stage, which involves conflicts in and of itself. The conductor invited two members to enter the playing space and chose the *duet* theatrical form, which creates conflict and is appropriate to the differentiation stage that the group was experiencing. The two members represented the different voices in the conflict, expressing the wish for safety, a home and a safe space versus the wish for self-expression and growth. They presented voices that expressed anxiety around accidents and mishaps, fear of growth (related to the tree and, perhaps, the process) and the fear of cracks appearing in one's safe space. The playing members expressed these voices while standing back to back, so that each voice had its own separate existence. Later on, the group engaged in a sharing circle, in which members reacted to the story and shared the materials that surfaced during the session.

When the conductor gathered up these different materials, he was able to reflect back to the group various themes related to the group process – how will the group be able to create a safe space – a home for everyone – that allowed members to grow; how will this group home be able to hold accidents and overflowing; how will we be able to handle ruptures and crises and support each other vis-à-vis the decisions we make and how will we be able to create a home that one could live in over time, on one's path to development and growth. As mentioned, the theatrical form served to heighten the discord between these voices, allowing for differentiation and even conflict. In the sharing circle, the group discussed their ability to reconcile these voices and contain them side by side.

In the group's 17th session, a family story was introduced into the group. Sue told the group about her father, who had been ill for about two years. The entire family had to care for him, while also taking care of her aging mother. For the children, taking care of their parents was a burden and heavy load and they were confronted with very complex situations. A. spoke angrily about her sister, who refused to shoulder the burden and share it, like all the other siblings. This situation drove A. and her sister apart, accentuating the gap between their relationship during the last year and how close they used to be.

In this case, the conductor chose to use a theatrical form called *talking heads*: three members stand side by side; in turn, each of them takes a step toward the audience and delivers a monologue for one of the story's characters. The three playing members chose to present the voices of the teller, her father and her sister. This allowed the introduction of a variety of perspectives about the story into the playing space: one performer reflected the experience of the teller and the other playing members echoed other perspectives. Some voices stressed the similarity between the different characters, while others attested to the difference between them. This form corresponds with the *mutuality* stage, in which members acknowledge the uniqueness of each voice in the group as well as the potential for development that lies in the gap between self and other. At this stage, criticism and conflict facilitate growth toward deepening one's closeness and intimacy with others and assuming responsibility over one's relationships.

When the theatrical response was over, Sue shared the insights that surfaced as she was listening to the various perspectives on the events that took place, especially her sister's perspective. She realized that her sister was able to present a position that existed within her as well – except that she was having difficulty expressing it: the frustration, the heavy load, the wish to shirk one's responsibility and simply look on from the sidelines. Sue shared that she felt a certain discomfort while watching the final scene of the theatrical response. The way the members were standing at the end manifested the distance between the two sisters whereas, at that point of the process, Sue was feeling a sense of recognition, acceptance of the different ways in which she and her sister were dealing with the situation and a wish for closeness.

The conductor turned to the playing members and asked them to use movement to represent the wish for closeness and mutual acceptance that Sue has just expressed. The members who played the two sisters positioned themselves in the playing space and created a movement with their hands and their gazes which emphasized that wish for intimacy between the two sisters, their yearning for one another and each sister's unique voice in relation to their father, who was also represented in the playing space by a third member. The talking heads form served to highlight the potential for growth toward greater intimacy and a deeper relationship, toward a place where each sister was bringing her unique personality to bear on her way of dealing with this intricate situation.

Note

1 This chapter is a revised version of a paper published by Keisari, Raz et al. (2018).

Chapter 9

Approaching personal stories through dramatic resonances in group work

Susana Pendzik

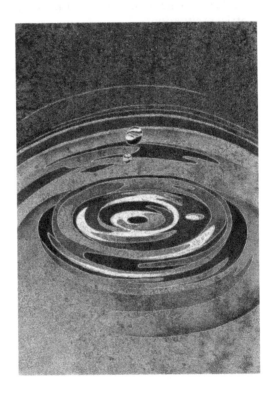

Figure 9.1 Resonances

The word "resonance" (from Latin *resonantia*) indicates an "echo" – a sound that is heard again (re-sonates). In music, it refers to the prolongation or reinforcement of a sound "by a vibrating body (*resonator*) attached to or in close proximity to the source of the sound" (Apel & Daniel, 2013, p. 245). In physics it denotes a phenomenon in which a vibration is produced within

DOI: 10.4324/9781003167822-10

a system in response to an external stimulus. In sympathetic resonance, "a specific frequency or sound wave will set in motion the same frequency in another object when they come into contact" (Kossak, 2015, p. 99). In psychotherapy, the notion has been linked to concepts such as "embodied empathy" (Sletvold, 2015), "affect attunement" and "emotional synchrony" – as it happens between mother and baby (Stern, 2002) (Fig. 9.1).

Dramatic resonances is a drama therapy-based approach, grounded in the transformative power of dramatic reality and its ability to produce resonances in the human psyche. The approach draws on the creative-intuitive responses of group members or the therapist to an "input" presented to them. The input may be a personal experience, issue, memory or dream, brought up by a participant or client, or a non-personal source (such as a myth, story, or literary text) introduced as a therapeutic intervention. The approach combines elements from various fields, among others, the shamanic paradigm and playback theater, mindfulness and intersubjectivity. This chapter describes the approach as applied in connection to a personal input in group therapy.

Dramatic reality as a therapeutic resonator

Dramatic reality is the concrete manifestation of human imagination in the here and now. Its presence characterizes all drama-based approaches to therapy, as the concrete embodiment of an "as if" world which is at the core of all dramatic interactions. Any therapist using drama as a tool engages with this concept (and to a great extent, other creative arts therapists as well). The influence of dramatic reality on therapeutic processes has been extensively reviewed in drama therapy and related fields literature (Blatner, 2000; Boal, 1995; Duggan & Grainger, 1997; Jennings, 1998; Johnson, 2009; Moreno, 1987; Pendzik, 2006; Pitruzzella, 2004; Winnicott, 2005).

Dramatic reality can be conceived as a potential *resonator*: As the contents of a therapeutic session are brought into contact with this realm, a subtle and intricate process of oscillation, destabilization, reorganization and transformation of old patterns is set into motion (Pendzik, 2006). A therapeutic interaction with dramatic reality detonates a dynamic – usually enjoyable – range of possibilities, which resonate in the psyche. As Boal (1995) claims, the aesthetic space (a synonym of dramatic reality) possesses a plasticity that liberates the imagination and a reflexive quality that makes it possible to observe it. In this space, the psyche is able to "resonate with the widest possible register" (Gersie and King, 1990, p. 333), therefore allowing for new meanings to be accepted or integrated by the mind.

As a resonator, dramatic reality can be used in different ways – each one producing a different kind of resonance. If we imagine dramatic reality as a drum, a person may play it and generate resonances between the sounds produced by the drum and his or her body; or someone else may play it and create a synchronous resonance in the instrument, the player and the listener. The same occurs in drama therapy: An input brought into dramatic reality elicits a resonance in the client, the therapist and/or the group.

Although in drama therapy both client and therapist may go in and out of dramatic reality, many approaches assume that the therapeutic benefit for the client comes primarily from personally inhabiting the "as if." However, in some approaches, clients resonate with dramatic reality as "spectators." One such instance is playback theater, in which conductors typically stand in the doorway, serving as a bridge between teller, audience and performers (Fox, 1994), while "tellers" partake from the event by watching it from the side (Salas, 2009). Similar formats are found in therapeutic storytelling or ritual performances, as well as in some therapeutic theater productions in which the "source" (the person providing the input) witnesses his/her experiences as performed by others (Ali et al., 2018; Hodermarska et al., 2016; Ray & Pendzik, 2021). The effectiveness of these approaches is based on theater's ability to generate an altered state of consciousness in the person, "whose distance from the drama supports a state of receptivity... [in which] ...the client becomes the witness" (Johnson, 1996, p. 116), as well as provides a measure of aesthetic distance that encourages self-reflection and resonance (Wood, 2018). In the "client as witness" intervention, a particular sort of resonance is promoted, which may be associated to the shamanic paradigm in drama therapy.

The shamanic paradigm in drama therapy and playback theater

Shamanism is a cross-cultural phenomenon found in human civilization since ancient times, in which healing and performance are bound together. It is assumed to be the foundation of theater and the arts (Schechner, 2005), reminding us that theater is inherently linked to *therapeusis*. As a culture-bound tradition, shamanism takes different forms. However, a prevailing idea is the ecstatic journey of the shaman who travels to non-ordinary reality to perform a mission on behalf of a community or a person: The shaman's journey is performed with the purpose of fighting a disease, restoring a lost soul, gathering information about the field, the river, life cycles, etc. (Eliade, 1972). As the journey through other cosmic regions proceeds, the landscape of the region, the beings encountered and the events experienced by the shaman become manifest through performative means, before the eyes of the client and/or audience. According to Cole (1975),

> Once arrived in the other world... [the shaman] uses mime to transmit back to his onlookers the adventures he is, psychically, having there: battles against divine animals or demons, social contacts with gods. The latter often gives rise to dialogues, in which the shaman speaks for both himself and the deity. The shaman must be something of an expert

in vocal characterization, for in the course of one of these dialogues he may be called upon to produce everything from the sounds of a horse drinking to the hiccups of a god. In addition to mime and dialogue, the shaman may draw on such incidental performance skills as ventriloquism and puppetry to help render his adventures in the other world.

(p. 19)

The shamanic tradition does not belong to a "primitive" past or to "exotic" cultures (from a Western point of view): it is a dynamic phenomenon that continues "to shape many people's personal, social, and/or cosmological identities today" (Zarrilli, 2006, p. 15). Moreover, as a conceptual paradigm, shamanism permeates any psychotherapeutic method that adopts the idea of rendering an embodied journey to "other worlds" – another metaphor for the "unconscious" – through performative means. Drama therapy, as well as other creative arts therapies, belongs to this category (Casson, 2016; Kim & Mastnak, 2015; Moreno, 2016; Pendzik, 1988, 2004, 2018; Snow, 2009). The shamanic ancestry is quite evident in approaches where the notion of "the client as witness" prevails, in which the shaman holds the process by acting as the client's representative in the "world beyond," voicing and embodying the client's needs and hopes like a "symbolic avatar."

Playback theater is clearly informed by the shamanic paradigm. Like shamans, who download the other world through performance, playback performers embark on a journey "on behalf of" the teller, enacting what they believe might be going on in their minds and hearts. The journey takes place in a context in which the client's safety is maintained through a set of culture-related rituals that make sense to the audience (Floodgate, 2006; Pendzik, 2008, 2018; Rowe, 2007), transforming lived experiences into well-crafted pieces of art that resonate with the teller and the audience (Salas, 2009).

Dramatic resonances: the approach

In an exercise reported by Gersie and King (1990) a Jewish woman shared with the group a childhood memory of not being allowed to have a Christmas tree by her parents. For some time, her parents let her have a tiny little tree in her room and adorn it only with homemade decorations, until one day her father told her that it was time to give it up. Group members were instructed to create mnemonic drawings inspired by this memory, sharing with her a part of the story that resonated with them. The woman was quite surprised to find out that some participants had given a lot of prominence to her father in the story, while she had felt that his role was just a functional one. The writers conclude that

not only did she become aware of how her memory appeared to other people and the impact it had on them, her attention was drawn to an alternative way of looking at the experience which until then had been inaccessible to her.

(p. 334)

This illustration exemplifies how the resonances work in a creative arts therapy context.

In a previous paper, I illustrated the idea of dramatic resonances using the image of throwing a stone into a quiet lake (Pendzik, 2008): The initial input is the stone, and the resonances are the ripples that follow. The ripples echo the input, generating a chain of patterns that create a wider shape – a unique gestalt, as reflected in the image by nature photographer, Fruma Markowitz (Figure 9.2). The input is what a person brings to therapy or supervision; the lake is dramatic reality. The resonances are the creative responses that the group or the therapist generates around that input from within dramatic reality. The responses are not verbal: they are artistically crafted and/or performed. Dramatic resonances seek to expand the original input through an artistic movement composed of aesthetic pulses (the resonances). The approach is aesthetically and therapeutically attuned.

Anyone who has observed the shapes created by something thrown into a calm lake knows that ripple shapes do not repeat themselves. Nature is the best teacher to learn about the aesthetics of resonances. A sequence of

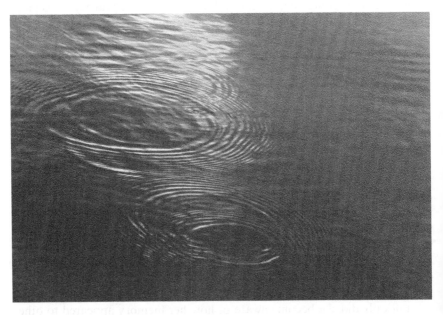

Figure 9.2 Fruma Markowitz Photo: Ripples in the water.

dramatic resonances may be improvised or rehearsed (even over several sessions) and can include, as an example, a pantomimed duet between protagonist and antagonist, the inner monologue of a character in the story, a familiar song that echoes it, a retelling of the story as if told to the narrator's yet-to-come grandchildren, a myth that embraces the input, and so on. The resonances are presented as a single performance, in attunement with the aesthetic flow they generate on stage.

Figure 9.3 presents a schematic picture of various categories of resonances, each positioned at a different aesthetic distance from the input. A resonance may *highlight* an aspect of the input (such as the emotional tone or the connection between characters); it may present a special angle by switching the *point of view* of the narrator, presenting the perspective of secondary characters or non-characters; it may *expand* the storyline, for example, by suggesting a scene that took place before the narrative began or by inventing its aftermath ("Ten years have passed since X and Y got married... how does their relationship look like today?"). *Framing* resonances can be used to place the input in a broader context, like a zoom-out shot. For instance, the input could be regarded as a scene from a movie or an excerpt that someone wrote in his personal diary, moving the focus to the broader context. In *personal resonances* the participants share a private experience that is analogous to the input. *Universal resonances* embrace the input through an

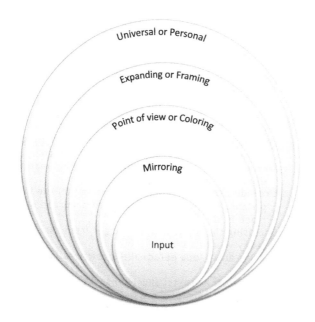

Figure 9.3 Classic Varieties of Dramatic resonances.

intertextual quote (a song or a proverb, for example) or through a universal story or myth. Table 9.1 describes the basic idea of each resonance type. The list is not exhaustive but exemplifies a variety of classic resonances that may be created vis-à-vis the input.

Dramatic resonances are not free associations: they are more akin to the Jungian than to the Freudian method for working with dreams (Fontana, 1997). While the latter encourages people to pay attention to the first association that arises in their mind and pursue the chain of thoughts that evolves from it, the Jungian approach encourages returning to the source after each association. While free associations advance as a chain, in the Jungian approach, the associations revolve around a central word or image that emerges from the dream, maintaining direct contact with it. Dramatic resonances are closer to Jung's idea because they stay in touch with the original input. Like the ripples in the lake, even as they move away, they continue to keep in touch with the input and to revolve around it.

To use Grotowski's terminology (1968), a resonance is an encounter between performers and witnesses, a meeting place between the input provider and the resonators. Except for the first ripple (mirror resonance), which tries to stay close to the source and reflect it faithfully, the more distant resonances express primarily what the input has elicited in other people. Thus, the input provider can witness the resonances without feeling obliged to accept them as interpretations or advice. In this sense, the method is analogous to the psychodramatic sharing circle, where group members are invited to express after the psychodrama "in what way the enactment reminded them of aspects of their own lives" (Blatner, 2000, p. 5). However, compared

Table 9.1 Dramatic resonances short definitions

Mirroring	Close to the text; a relatively faithful representation of the input.
Highlighting	Emphasizing a certain aspect of the narration, such as the emotional tone, the dynamics between characters.
Point of view	Playing with the focus on characters; illuminating non-dominant or unusual perspectives.
Expanding	Extending the narrative (before or after) the input; set; potential scenes that could have occurred or may take place in the future.
Framing	Enclosing the input within a larger framework (zoom-out, story within a story).
Personalizing	Sharing analogous personal experiences in an aesthetic way.
Intertextual or universal resonances	Quoting other texts; allusive parallel creations (songs, poems, proverbs); connecting the input with archetypal sources (myths, universal narratives, natural phenomena).

to the sharing in psychodrama (which closes the dramatic action and is usually done verbally), dramatic resonances come after the initial input (usually verbal) and are always presented from within dramatic reality.

Using dramatic resonances as a group therapy technique

When used in this format, dramatic resonances involve the creative responses of group participants to a personal story or issue put forth by one of its members. The technique consists of four steps: (a) presenting the input; (b) creating a mirror resonance; (c) developing additional resonances; (d) performing the resonances as aesthetically organized vignettes.

Presenting the input

The technique has a ceremonial character: The initial input is conceived as a kind of "offering" presented within the "sacred space" of the group. In order to create the appropriate atmosphere, the group is first led through a series of grounding exercises aimed at encouraging concentration, introspection and connection. Techniques derived from mindfulness (Kabat-Zinn, 1994) and meditative movement practices – such as authentic movement (Pallaro, 1999) – are used to help create the group container, fostering active listening and intersubjectivity.

Participants are instructed to listen to the input while remaining open and alert to feelings and emotions, images, symbols and stories that resonate with them as they witness the input. The input is conveyed as a monologue or as a solo, marking its beginning and end with the sound of a musical instrument or another ritualistic means.

The mirror resonance

This resonance is vital in a therapeutic setting, for the narrator needs to experience a resonance that is as close as possible to the "text" they chose to share. Many psychotherapy schools consider the "mirror" to be a crucial stage in early human development (Kohut, 1984; Kohut & Wolf, 1978; Lacan, 1984; Rogers, 1986). Consequently, "mirroring" is a significant therapeutic intervention in a variety of approaches, including drama therapy and psychodrama (Emunah, 2020; Johnson, 2009; Moreno, 1987). Whether mirroring is done with the Rogerian aim of helping clients to be self-empowered through "unconditional positive regard" or, as Kohut claims, as a necessary developmental milestone on the road to the resolution of the transference, the input-presenter needs to feel heard, to be assured that the group has listened to their story fully and empathetically and that they understand the experience from his/her perspective.

The tendency to skip this stage often elicits feelings of frustration, lone-liness or social isolation in the narrator – an experience that is inconsist-ent with the therapeutic spirit of drama therapy and playback theater (Fox, 1994; Salas, 2009). Quite a few times I witnessed situations in which there was not enough "sticking to the text" of a teller, moving instead too soon, too far, from the person's experience. For instance:

> A university student shared in a playback theatre group his being over-whelmed during the period of exams, which reminded him of childhood experiences in school, in which he had various somatic reactions to test-related stress. The actor that began the playback performance cre-ated a scene involving a child that had been diagnosed ADHD (some-thing that was never mentioned in the student's account of the facts), and somehow the whole piece ended up revolving around this mistaken diagnosis. The teller was too shy at the time (and also confused) to say that the representation was inaccurate, so he left feeling bitter and mis-understood. Only a few weeks later, he was able to share his disappoint-ment and hurt for being misinterpreted.

While it is true that in an ongoing therapeutic group this "empathic failure" (Kohut & Wolf, 1978) could potentially become a repairing experience, the ideal path is for the person to feel secure and contained by the group so that further resonances can also "do the work" of bringing the voice of alter-ity into the picture. I call this phenomenon the "wounded teller effect" – a teller who feels betrayed, helpless and lonely, after exposing personal experi-ences in a milieu that promised, and did not deliver, empathic listening. The mirror resonance offers the input provider a basic experience of trust, after which it becomes easier to be more open to the transformations elicited by subsequent resonances. In addition, the mirror resonance gives group mem-bers a chance to step into the narrator's shoes and experience empathy, thus gaining their "right" to transform the content and spiral it onto a different ripple of the lake.

Augusto Boal (1995) distinguishes between three types of empathic rela-tions that an actor may develop toward an aesthetic image represented on stage, which express different degrees of responsiveness. These are identi-fication, recognition and resonance. Identification is the closest type: An actor-participant identifies with a situation when it evokes a similar per-sonal experience. Recognition takes place when an individual can relate to a situation, not through a personal experience, but "second hand," through a close person: "I know exactly what this person is talking about because it happened to my father..." Resonance is the third degree in terms of dis-tance; it presents a situation that "sounds familiar" even though neither I nor anyone close to me went through something similar. According to Boal

(1995), although all three types are valuable points of departure, resonance allows for the discovery of hidden aspects, perhaps precisely because it is experienced as a more diffused type of resemblance.

We may say, in the spirit of Boal's ideas, that the mirror resonance is similar to the identification state, in which group members are invited – and challenged – to express first-degree identifications with the input. As a response performed immediately after the input is offered, the mirror resonance cannot convey a vague likeness or personal associations of group members to the situation presented – such as the ADHD interpretation of the actor mentioned above. Perhaps mirroring can be related to the universal pleasure derived from of "mimesis," as asserted by Aristotle in the *Poetics*: "the reason why ... [people] enjoy seeing a likeness is, that in contemplating it they find themselves learning or inferring, and saying perhaps, 'Ah, that is he.'" (2008, p. 6). Indeed, both aesthetic and affective ingredients may account for the pleasure of mimesis (Pitruzzella, 2017), which may explain the need for the mirror resonance as a point of departure in the dramatic resonance method.

Simple techniques can be used (like playback theater short forms) that illustrate the input rather mimetically, with the understanding, of course, that the lake is not an accurate mirror but a subjective one. Here are two techniques that illustrate a mirror resonance.

- The image technique (from Boal's (1995) Image Theatre). A picture of the input is presented in the form of a static group sculpture, consisting of several participants (not necessarily all the group), which reproduces the input as a composition. It may be "brought to life" for a few seconds, through movement and sound images that strictly reflect the input. This technique can also be applied with inputs that have several scenes, in which case, various images can be produced.

  A group member refers an experience of getting lost in a forest at night. Four players create a still image in which the protagonist is sitting on the floor, holding her head with her hands with frightened look in her eyes, and three participants stand as "tall trees" with their backs toward her and their eyes closed or covered. The sculpture comes to life for some moments, conveying the wind and a few night-bird sounds.

- The "cut-and-paste chorus" resembles a playback chorus composed of three to four group members, who are instructed to only use the words, sentences and gestures that were pronounced in the input, albeit in a different order and playing with intonations. Each word or phrase that a chorus member says is repeated at least twice by other participants. The chorus is instructed to keep an eye on how the piece begins and ends, in order to create an aesthetic experience for the input giver.

Developing resonances: spiraling onto other ripples

After a brief processing with the narrator for feedback and comments, the group is invited to let other resonances unfold. The narrator usually does not participate in the group resonances (unless the process extends beyond one session), but receives another task from the facilitator, such as creating a personal resonance that allows some quality time and private reflection. Instructions given to the narrator range from writing or drawing something about the input or processing the mirror resonance, to going for a walk nearby, looking for a stone that symbolizes the input or finding a title for the performance that they are about to witness. These guidelines maintain the narrator in a kind of liminal space, which contains great transformative and therapeutic potential (Blatner, 2000; Turner,1982). The premise is that the narrator is not yet ripe to return to the collective space where they will be required to take an active role in the deconstruction of the input, deal with the group dynamics, ponder over aesthetic dilemmas and so on. Instead, staying in the liminal space prepares the input-provider to open up to the resonances that the group will offer and let the experience of the "client as witness" resonate within.

The resonances are a series of creative vignettes that deconstruct the initial input into short aesthetic beats. They can be planned or improvised. If the group is new or unfamiliar with the technique, the facilitator may offer participants specific options for resonances, helping them to create small teams to develop a variety of ideas. In a group with experience in the technique, participants can declare what kinds of resonances they want to prepare, gathering in teams to work around these ideas. Another possibility is to open the stage to "spontaneous resonances" – i.e., a round of impromptu resonances. A group performing spontaneous resonances has to be familiar with the method's guiding rules. These include, for example, that the initiator of a resonance has a grip on its "vision," so that other group members may join in the scene, but the leading role and the responsibility to bring the vignette to an end belong to the initiator. Also, emphasis is placed on the awareness of timing and aesthetics, whereby members have to keep in mind the appropriateness and timeliness of their offers.

Using the degree of guidance that the group needs, and in consultation with the participants, the facilitator lets group members make the aesthetic and therapeutic choices intuitively and collectively, or alternatively, suggests a structure for the resonances. Listening to the pace and the timing of the group is essential. A skilled group can look back when the final resonance is over and discover a significant aesthetic structure. While it is not always possible to define these patterns in words, they can be perceived as they are in an artistic creation, the opening of a flower or the sequence of a dream. "Aesthetic choices" are not only a matter of personal taste. As Susan Langer (1953) argues, the common feature of all works of art, regardless of the culture or civilization to which they belong, is their ability to mold meaningful contents in shapes that evoke "aesthetic feelings." Here is an example of a full sequence:

A young researcher relates an experience of sexual harassment by a public figure who was the guest of honor at a conference in which she had been requested by the academic committee to assist him during his stay. The experience was confusing as his advances were mostly performed in public and seemingly done in "good humor." In one instance he introduced her to one of his colleagues at a cocktail party by distorting a private matter she had shared with him earlier, giving a sexual connotation to it. Although the comment had caused embarrassment, the woman had kept silent and did not do anything at the time, being left with feelings of guilt, humiliation and anger.

> The mirror resonance involved a still picture of the scene with the three characters at the cocktail party, focusing on the expressions of their faces. The input-giver was offered to paint a picture evoked by the experience, while three teams worked on resonances: The first resonance presented monologues by the two men at the party, in which the guest of honor was ostensibly unaware of doing anything "wrong", and his colleague felt ashamed, thinking that this young researcher could have been his own daughter, and feeling mortified for not having reacted (point of view). Another resonance took the case to a "me-two" court, presenting a scene located in a potential future, in which many women complain about this public figure (expanding). The last resonance revolved around the Greek myth of Philomela, raped by her brother-in-law Tereus, who also cut her tongue to keep her silent. However, Philomela wove a tapestry depicting the story, and thus made it known (universal resonance). The presentation ended with a spontaneous resonance in which a member added a "moral" to the myth linking the teller's academic research to Philomela's tapestry, and encouraging women and men to make these experiences public.

At the end of the resonance sequence there is usually a verbal processing, although silence is also welcome. Like the processing in drama therapy, this verbal processing is mainly aimed at integrating the experiences of both the presenters and the witness (narrator). Surely, the input elicit contents that may need processing, but the course of the work itself also reflects group issues and receives reference. The aesthetic choices of the group are talked about, and the participants share their reflections on the choices made, in the general form of the resonances, in the gestalt created. In summary there is an attempt to integrate verbally the different levels of the experience: personal, interpersonal, group and aesthetic.

Therapeutic and aesthetic considerations, such as "aesthetic distance" (Landy, 1996), are contemplated when using dramatic resonances. Holding the pulse of the group, the facilitator may ask participants which resonance can open or close the sequence. In the following example with an experienced group, the narrator, Dora (pseudonym), a woman over 60 years old, shared a painful experience of losing her daughter in a car accident.

Despite the fact that more than twenty years had passed since the event, the memory resurfaced with great force when two of her grandchildren got to the same age as her daughter was at the time of the accident. She evoked the events of the accident, the summer night, the moon, the vehicle speeding down a village street, the despair, the great loss... She then described how, for the first few months, she used to go to the accident site at night, screaming at the cars to lower their speed, shouting that there are children around.

Four group members performed a cut-and-paste chorus (see above) as a mirror resonance. This was very moving for the narrator, and she was instructed to write a journal entry, while the group elaborated the resonances.

The group developed the following resonances: The first resonance was the myth of Demeter and her daughter Persephone, showing Demeter's mourning of the disappearance of her daughter by wandering the earth in search for her, day and night, with torches (universal resonance). Then the moment of the car accident was acted in movement and sound (no words), in slow motion (highlighting), following which, monologues by the car and the moon on the night of the accident were presented (point of view). A scene in the future showing Dora having a good relationship with her grandchildren. However, the ghost of the accident appears in Dora's head, but the grandchildren see it and end up defeating it with the power of imagination and play (expanding). Finally, two group members intertwined personal experiences that resonated with Dora's story: a son who died shortly after birth, and a daughter who overcame a serious illness.

The session ended with a verbal processing. The group in general commented that the work around Dora's story had moved very deep emotions, generating a sense of cohesion. Dora was grateful that they have been able to contain such a heavy input – that it is almost unmentionable. She said that the resonance of Demeter was very touching, and that it was also reassuring that her grandchildren helped her to overcome the ghost. The therapist asked her to give a title to the piece. Dora named it after her daughter.

In this session, the cut-and-paste mirror resonance evoked a chorus of mourners. Although normally a sequence of resonances would begin with ripples that are closer to the original input, in this case, the opening resonance alluded to the myth of Demeter and Persephone, which was both an aesthetic derivative of the mirror resonance and a group need. The group felt it was right to distance from the personal level and start with a universal story that would provide collective support to the experience. Indeed, the decision to begin the resonance sequence with the myth turned out to be a successful aesthetic choice that served both the group and the narrator in the construction of a good group container. This container is the intersubjective space where the resonances take place. As Hammer (2015) describes it, in an intersubjective relationship one relates to the other with what feels subjectively most real to oneself and what one senses to be subjectively most real to the other. In his words, "if someone goes into a store and asks for a container of milk, that is interpersonal; but if he senses that the clerk feels depressed and says something supportive to cheer him, then that is intersubjective" (p. 92).

Summary and conclusions

An ability to generate resonances requires first of all the development of good listening skills and the capacity to communicate. In order to elaborate resonances a person needs to be open to the other, and, simultaneously, well connected to their own process. This is why practicing the technique has in itself a therapeutic value (Pendzik, 2008). If we compare again dramatic resonances to free associations, in associations one says, "this is what the issue your brought up evokes in me," thus shifting the focus from the experience source to that of the listener. Free associations usually throw us into our inner world, which may not necessarily resonate with the world or the imagination of others. Resonances require additional effort of empathy and communication because the goal is to make at least two entities resonate. Resonances have meaning for others besides myself; they contain within an intersubjective response that includes the "other."

Dramatic resonances is an advanced therapeutic intervention that uses the collective to assist the individual and the group. The technique provides a protected container where participants can practice and develop positive interpersonal relationships and intersubjectivity while cultivating their inner artist (Pendzik, 2008). The approach facilitates an exchange of narratives, anchoring the personal experience in the collective realm. Many ego functions are mobilized through the practice of the technique, hence one of its limitations: When dramatic resonances are practiced in full format, as presented in the chapter, they require emotional maturity, cognitive abilities and social adjustment. You need a calm and peaceful lake in order to throw a stone that will create significant resonances for someone else. Practicing the technique in its full scale may be difficult with some populations. As a start, people may need to develop basic skills in order to experience an "inner lake" through mindfulness and embodiment exercises, which should not prevent the therapist from trying to build these resources. Although the method has been explored primarily as a group approach, dramatic resonances can also be adapted to individual work, as well as constitute a valuable tool in supervision and training in drama therapy and other therapeutic modalities.

Chapter 10

Psychotherapeutic Playback Theater as a group dream about the story

Surrealism as the theatrical language of the inner world

Ronen Kowalsky, Nir Raz, Shoshi Keisari

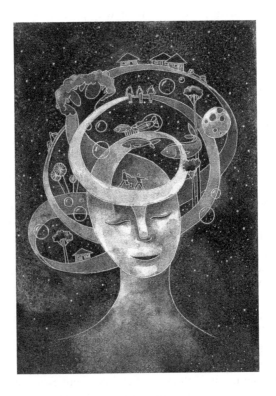

Figure 10.1

The literal meaning of the term *surrealism* is "beyond reality": it is a combination of the French words *sur*, meaning above or beyond, and *realism*, meaning the faithful representation of reality. The term refers to art that goes "beyond the real" in an attempt to offer an introspective glance into

DOI: 10.4324/9781003167822-11

the human psyche. Surrealism draws its material from the inner world and uses dream language, images, symbols, the unconscious and the imagination as sources of artistic inspiration. It often entails the irrational and the surprising. This artistic movement is mostly associated with visual artists such as Salvador Dali, Rene Magritte and Juan Miro. In this chapter, which concludes the book, we will explore the development of the surrealist movement in various art forms and the ways in which this movement can inspire creative processes in Psychotherapeutic Playback Theater.

The surrealist movement in visual arts and theater

The surrealist movement was founded by André Breton (1969), who published the surrealist manifesto in 1924. This movement emerged in response to the bleak state of the world in the wake of the First World War, which left people feeling that order and reason have failed. Surrealism, which sought to represent freedom and liberation from the chains of war and the regimes that led to such unprecedented death and devastation, rebelled against contemporary aesthetic conventions by introducing randomness, absurdity and unbridled creativity. Surrealist artists were also deeply influenced by the ideas of Sigmund Freud regarding the unconscious and the language of dreams as direct means of communication with the unconscious parts of the psyche.

One of the pioneers of surrealist theater is Antonin Artaud (1896–1948), a French actor, playwright and theoretician who played a major role in the development of modern Western theater. Artaud's approach, which profoundly changed the nature of theater in the second half of the 20th century, sought to undermine the conventions of realistic theater and replace it with a mythical, physical and visual theater. The goal of this new theater was to promote social and political changes and even offer a new notion of the human mind. Artaud's "inner world" theater positioned itself in surreal, dreamlike spaces and attempted to present the world of images and internal experiences unencumbered by the realistic layers that obfuscate it. His most influential theoretical work is *The Theater and Its Double* (Artaud, 1958), whose key notion is manifest in its paradoxical title, seeing as it is theater which is often perceived as reality's "double." In this essay, Artaud argues for the creation of a theater that will render reality its own double – a theater exploring the general pattern which creates each individual life as a particular manifestation thereof. To this end, Artaud looked for various means of expressing the language of the inner world on stage.

Resembling Artaud's artistic outlook, Psychotherapeutic Playback Theater seeks to express theatrically the myriad voices of the inner world and the various shades and perspectives to which it gives rise. To achieve this purpose, group members in Psychotherapeutic Playback Theater need, much like surrealist artists, to create their theatrical response in the language of dreams. The theatrical response in Psychotherapeutic Playback Theater can, to a great extent, be viewed as a group dream about the story. The conductor can instruct members, while they are listening to the story, to imagine it as a dream. The purpose of such an instruction is for the listening members to perceive the story not merely realistically, taking it at face value, but as an expression of the teller's inner world. In order to make the transition from the realistic story to the surrealistic inner world, one must engage in the process of observation through "free floating attention." "Loosening the screws" and "seeing the story at a lower resolution" are some of the metaphors that come up in the group in relation to this process and that can serve the conductor in guiding the group to re-envision the story as a dream.

Bion (1962), followed by Ogden (2003), framed therapy in terms of rehabilitating the person's ability to create dream-thoughts; not to become mired in the tangle of reality's concrete details but to free one's capacity for creative thinking and soar beyond these. According to Bion and Ogden, mental difficulties emerge when this ability has been lost due to a traumatic event that left a kind of scar on one's psychic tissue. Just as a physical scar prevents the flow of blood and oxygen, a psychic scar limits the extent of aliveness and movement that imbue one's thoughts and experiences. In order to illustrate the techniques and methods that cultivate the members' surrealist mindset, we will examine the three surrealist movements of the plastic arts and their historical development: automatism, figurative surrealism and abstract surrealism.

Automatism

Automatism in art seeks to create a state in which the artist relinquishes all pre-existing knowledge, value systems and cultural background and avoids any pre-planning of their creation, in order to facilitate intuitive action. This movement urges artists to refrain from following any aesthetic, logic or narrative considerations and instead draw on their individual, even idiosyncratic associative capacity as the highway to the psychic world. They should thus be engaged in the artistic expression of unconscious material. In the surrealist manifesto, Breton (1969) argues in favor of direct action, free of any pre-planning, which automatically bursts onto the canvas or the page. In his words:

> Psychic automatism in its pure state, by which one proposes to express – verbally, by means of the written word, or in any other manner – the actual functioning of thought. Dictated by thought, in the absence of any control exercised by reason, exempt from any aesthetic or moral concern.
>
> (p. 26)

Automatism seeks to unravel familiar patterns – whether narrative or otherwise – and encourage an associative flow that is unbound by limits and rules. It even attempts to undo technical patterns, by neutralizing the natural tendencies of the eye and the hand. This has led to the development of certain approaches that encourage the practice of automatic writing with one's off hand, which is unaccustomed to writing. In the realm of theater, automatism in manifest in the form of improvised and intuitive theatrical action. Certain elements and influences originating in the automatism movement can be noted in Psychotherapeutic Playback Theater, namely, in the willingness, during fully spontaneous (open) improvisations, to enter the playing space without any pre-planning or clear ideas and in the unstructured work of open improvisation. These methods facilitate the emergence of spontaneous and intuitive occurrences in the playing space (keeping in mind the psychic significance of such work methods, as discussed throughout the book).

Jackson Pollock (1956–2012), who practiced "action painting," is a good example of the application of automatism in plastic art. In his view, the work of art lies in the action, rather than the end result. For this reason, his work process utilized large canvases, dripping and splashing techniques and dance movements. Various improvised works of art as well as certain stages in the process of Psychotherapeutic Playback Theater are greatly inspired by Pollock's paintings and serve as its visual analogues: a jumble of free associations that amount to a complete painting, whose recognizable aesthetic was achieved spontaneously and unintentionally. According to Pollock, the true essence of art is not the resulting product but the facilitation of psychic transformation through artistic action. We see this argument as the very foundation of the Psychotherapeutic Playback Theater process. In this context, we recall a saying by Maimonides: "As for the soul, the soul has no structure. It is the process" (2010, p. 16).

Figurative surrealism

Surrealist artists looked at the works they had created through automatic processes and discovered that they exhibit certain inherent and recurring aesthetic structures and figures. This type of observation led to the birth of the second surrealist movement – figurative surrealism. Artworks created by this movement present images that are composed of representations of realistic objects and part-objects, joined together in ways that are not bound to the laws of reason, resulting in a dreamlike syntax of images. Many of these works, including those of Rene Magritte (1898–1967) and Salvador Dali (1904–1989), make ample use of the recurrence of images, amplifying the emergent dreamlike feeling. Consider, for example, the following excerpt from a short story, "The Aleph," by Jorge Luis Borges:

> [...] Saw horses with wind-whipped manes on a beach in the Caspian Sea at dawn, saw the delicate bones of a hand, saw the survivors of a battle sending postcards, saw a Tarot card in a shop window in Mirzapur, saw the oblique shadows of ferns on the floor of a greenhouse, saw tigers, pistons, bisons, tides, and armies.
>
> (Borges, 1949/1998, p. 283)

Here, Borges is using one of his favorite techniques. By creating a catalog of unrelated descriptions, though none of the individual images are in any way "supernatural" or transcendent, the resulting impression is a kind of vague, uncanny and surreal cosmic convergence.

Freud (1899), followed by the surrealist artists, formulated the principles of primary thinking, the psychic process which governs the formation of dreams and the language of the inner world. According to Freud, dreams have their own inherent structure, language and rules. For example, the dream takes place in a continuous present, with no past or future, before or after, cause and effect. This present includes both the past and the future through a principle Freud calls "condensation" – the time and narrative of the dream are condensed into a kind of continuous present (Freud, 1899). The principle of *condensation* also applies to dream impressions of space and characters: places in dreams are actually several places compressed together and characters are a condensed amalgamation of different people. A single dream image can thus use condensation to simultaneously include both the past and the future within a single occurrence or several people from one's real life within a single dream character. Dreams also utilize the mechanism of *displacement,* by which threatening contents are transferred onto a neutral object, making it more accessible to the dreamer's mind. For example, a person who is terrified about losing their livelihood or their ability to work may dream about a bird with a broken wing, which cannot fly. Because the dream is lifelike and presents concrete objects that are things in themselves, these dream images are not experienced as such, but hold the emotional world displaced onto them on an experiential-concrete level. Finally, dreams, like surrealist art, also entail the principle of repetition, by which certain images recur and resurface in various forms.

Psychotherapy involves an attempt to rehabilitate the ability to create dream-thoughts by relating to the contents of a story, a conversation or an encounter as having the quality of a dream (Bion, 1962; Ogden, 2003). During a therapy session, one can observe various elements as containing hidden psychic materials, informing one's view of "regular" occurrences – such as the beginning of the session, the way the patient walks in the door or writes a check – as representing recurring psychic patterns which reveal something about that person. As seen later in this chapter, figurative surrealism greatly influenced Psychotherapeutic Playback Theater.

Abstract surrealism

The abstract surrealism movement begins with painter Juan Miro's (1893–1983) claim that figurative surrealism is too neatly organized. In his view, the contents of the inner world are naked sensory experiences, inherently devoid of any clearly figural representation. "Inner world" representations are essentially more sensorial, expressing qualities such as hotness or coldness, textures that conjure up physical sensations and colors, which also represent feelings and states of being. Miro led this abstract trend within surrealist art, promoting practices of hallucination-like painting, which draws on a uniquely individual and idiosyncratic formal idiom. This movement tends to paint objects in an abstract fashion, which is almost utterly unrelated to their actual appearance, resulting in objects that seems to be floating about in an indefinite space. Miro encouraged automatic painting, by which the artist allows the paintbrush to move freely across the canvas and only then looks at the emerging forms and lines and acknowledges the outcome as a work of art.

Following Winnicott (1949/1975), Ogden argues that the most basic levels of psychic experience take place in an essentially sensorial modality, in an experiential area where psyche and soma are yet indistinguishable (Ogden, 1989). He calls this area the *autistic-contiguous position* and argues that it is the locus of one-dimensional experiences that precede the splitting associated with Klein's (1975) paranoid-schizoid position. According to Winnicott (1949/1975) and Ogden (1989), any therapeutic process which does not engage this experiential level is partial at best and liable to leave the psyche's fundamental vulnerabilities unattended and unprocessed. In Psychotherapeutic Playback Theater, playing members are encouraged to engage in experiential-sensory-abstract work. The use of movement, cloths, music and voice amounts to an assortment of abstract elements, whose connection often exceeds the context of the original realistic narrative. This connection seeks to communicate directly with the inner world and express it experientially through theatrical creation. In this manner, the transformation of psychic material in the playing space is able to touch on the autistic-contiguous layer of experience, both that of the teller and those of the other members – the performers and the audience.

Surrealism in Psychotherapeutic Playback Theater

In the same vein as the surrealist artists, Psychotherapeutic Playback Theater seeks to create a theatrical image that captures the inner world. The use of surrealism allows for the creation of theater pieces that express psychic material in the psyche's native idiom and is, therefore, highly advisable in the theatrical responses of Psychotherapeutic Playback Theater. One of the basic principles of both surrealism and dream-work, which is also utilized in Psychotherapeutic Playback Theater, is that of condensation which, as mentioned, allows several elements, ideas or figures to exist simultaneously within a single image or occurrence. For example, the figure of a little girl who appears in a patient's dream can simultaneously be the patient herself as a child, the patient's daughter and a student from the class she teaches. Similarly, the figure of a little girl in Psychotherapeutic

Playback Theater can manifest the "girliness" of the story, which simultaneously transcends these figures and comprises them. A similar condensation of time, as mentioned above, takes place in both psychic space and Psychotherapeutic Playback Theater and allows for the conjunction (and even convergence) of different times and different characters, of events and mental states belonging to the past, the present or the future.

We will now present several principles of Psychotherapeutic Playback Theater which manifest surrealistic qualities in improvised theatrical work. These principles entail the processes of expansion and condensation, respectively, facilitating the expansion of reality beyond its realistic limits and the simultaneous co-existence of several elements within a single occurrence in the playspace.

These principles are illustrated through the use of surrealist dream-thoughts in five different reflections of a story told in a Psychotherapeutic Playback Theater group. Sonya, a 28-year-old woman, often shares with the group stories that involve a great deal of conflict. She talks about her great difficulty with making life choices and her somewhat obsessive preoccupation with the downsides and the costs of the choices she had made. In this context, she has told the group about her painful deliberation processes about moving out on her own, entering a romantic relationship and choosing what to study academically. Similarly, she said that, in the sessions, she often ended up not sharing her stories because, by the time she could decide what she wanted to tell, someone else was already sharing theirs. One session, after Sonya had not shared anything for a while, the conductor addressed her directly, asking if she wanted to share a story with the group. Sonya blushed and said, "I have a little something. I'm not sure if it's even a story that is suitable for playback. It's just a little something that happened to me at the store."

Sonya shared that, several days earlier, she went to the supermarket to buy groceries. When she got to the checkout counter, she noticed a strong, appetizing aroma coming from the store bakery. She was not sure whether she should leave the checkout counter halfway through her purchase and walk over to the bakery to buy that delicious freshly baked pastry. She felt uncomfortable just leaving and decided to simply continue her purchase. The cordial cashier lady said to her, "wow, something over at the bakery sure smells good, huh?" Sonya smiled and said, "I was thinking of going over and getting whatever it is that smells so good, but I felt bad about making people wait." The cashier winked at her and said, "it's fine, you can go ahead, and get a little something for me while you're at it." Sonya walked eagerly toward the store bakery, knowing that she has the cashier's approval. She followed the smell, which grew stronger and stronger as she approached the bakery. When she got there, she saw that the counter was empty. She decided not to give up and called out to the baker: "excuse me! Is there anyone here?" The baker, a man in his 70s stepped out to the counter and told her that a batch of large chocolate chip cookies just came out of the oven.

He was supposed to start packing them, but he would love to give her a few extra-fresh cookies. As usual, Sonya could not decide how many to get and eventually bought four cookies for herself and her boyfriend and another one for the cashier lady. On her way back to the checkout counter, Sonya could feel through the paper bag how hot the cookies were and imagined taking a bite and feeling the chocolate chips melt in her mouth. She was delighted that she was able to get the okay to pick up the cookies despite the growing line at the register.

When she got back to the register, the cashier noticed the bag of cookies and greeted Sonya with a big smile. She took the entire bag and put it somewhere behind her. Sonya felt very awkward. She already accepted having to give up the cookies because she did not want to get into an argument with the cashier, but then she felt her desire for the cookies stirring inside her, mixed with anger: "she took my cookies!" Sonya reached and grabbed the bag of cookies, took out one of them and said to the cashier lady with an apologizing smile: "you misunderstood. The cookies are for me. Only this one is for you." The cashier accepted the cookie with a scowl and, from that moment on, stopped being nice and genial toward Sonya. She checked out Sonya's items in an irritable silence, occasionally stopping to look at her phone. Sonya felt very uncomfortable and left the supermarket feeling ashamed and ill at ease. When she finally got home, she showed her boyfriend the bag of cookies with a smile and a sense of victory. He looked at the cookies and said, "thank you, sweetie, but I don't like this kind." Sonya went to the kitchen, made herself a cup of coffee and ate all four cookies in silence. They no longer tasted that good, maybe even a little bland.

Sonya's story is an example of a story whose therapeutic utilization requires re-envisioning in terms of dream-thoughts, which would shift it from the realm of the anecdotal and into the domain of the inner world. One could see the story as an invitation to contemplate its various elements (the cashier lady, the old baker, the cookies, Sonya's inner voices, etc.) as condensed symbols. In order to emphasize the conceptual elaboration required by the theatrical processing of this story, the conductor chose a partially planned improvisation, in which members were divided into several sub-groups. This form highlights and invites a variety of perspectives on the story, with each group choosing a single key idea to develop in its pre-planned improvisation. We will now demonstrate the application of several principles of surrealist thinking in Psychotherapeutic Playback Theater, through the exploration of different elements in the theatrical responses presented by the sub-groups in response to Sonya's story.

Moving between times and locations

Jacob Levy Moreno (1965) used the notion of *surplus reality* to stress that the dramatic process facilitates movement between times and places and even allows for the presentation of scenes that exist in one's inner world. Similarly, improvised theater pieces in Psychotherapeutic Playback Theater can simultaneously hold past, present and future. For example, the theatrical representation of the figure of the teller can converse with herself as a child – as the two figures are portrayed by two performers. This scene can be joined by yet another performer, who will portray the teller's future self and these three instances of the teller can then merge together or separate further. The possibility of simultaneously presenting different time dimensions – much like dream images – enables a profound exploration of psychic material.

This principle also involves the presentation of theatrical moments that combine several different places and times. For example, a character can move between countries – from a classroom in Romania to her present home in Israel and then back to Romania climbing a mountain with her father. All these can exist simultaneously in the playing space, just as they do in the dream. Transitions are easy and flexible and, while impossible in everyday concrete reality, they exhibit an internal logic that all members can understand.

The response presented by the first group in response to Sonya's story sought to highlight the element of childlike desire. They chose to portray the teller as a child playing "treasure hunt" with two other kids, looking for "the trove of lost cookies." The teller led the hunt and the two other children followed her, saying: "when we find the trove of lost cookies it would be amazing! We'd get to eat all the cookies we want!" They held a piece of paper in their hand – a "treasure map" – and underwent all kinds of adventures. On their quest, they fought the fire-breathing cashier-dragon and met the old baker who pointed them in the right direction. At some point during the hunt, they heard the voice of their mother calling: "come on home! It's getting late!" The children said goodbye and went away and the teller said, "We'll meet again tomorrow and continue our search for the trove of lost cookies. Maybe we'll find it someday." This version highlights a constant search for some lost object of desire as the core of the story. The fact that this object of desire is a kind of food stresses that the roots of this story are in the teller's childhood.

This version presents the quest for one's object of desire as an impossible goal, but in the process of hunting for it the children become friends and their relationship becomes a tangible, valuable achievement. The childhood memories of shared play become a treasure that one carries as an adult.

Personification of inner voices and emotional experiences

The theatrical image can offer a tangible embodiment of inner voices, presenting emotions, thoughts, wishes and dreams as concrete dramatic representations. Dali drew on what he termed "objectification" – the capacity to use art to transform an abstract concept or idea into a concrete object. This means that playing members can come in the playspace and physically embody characters such as "fear" or "hope." These roles are expressed through movements, gestures, spoken lines, music or voice in the process of reflecting the relevant aspects of the story and exploring the teller's inner world. These "inner-voice" characters have their own specific identity allowing the teller to acknowledge them and their intricacy. Thus, the representation of each particular element becomes distinct and clear for the playing members, the audience and the teller.

In the theatrical response presented by the second sub-group in response to Sonya's story, the figure of the teller entered the playspace blindfolded by a piece of cloth. All around her, at a certain distance, the other members moved about, each of them dancing with a different colored cloth. They called out her name several times – "come, Sonya... come, Sonya..." – embodying different objects of desire in her life. They started as the cookies and then expanded this idea to include the first guy she fell in love with, a trip she had wanted to take but ended up not taking, a place she wanted to live in. Another performer played the teller's guilty conscience: he repeatedly came between her figure and her objects of desire, chiding her – "this isn't right for you! Get your act together! This is no way to behave!" The figure of the teller moved toward the various voices who called out her name and, each time, the figure of the guilty conscience grabbed her by the shoulders and pulled her back to the center of the playing space.

This version posited the struggle between the desires of the id and the prohibitions of the super-ego as the heart of the story. It emphasized the dilemma concerning which voice led Sonya's actions and the feeling of walking through dark, unknown and uncontrollable areas. It is a powerful expression of Sonya's experience of being emotionally torn between these voices and of her wish to integrate them.

Simultaneous portrayal of multiple dramatic roles

As mentioned, theatrical response can contain several representations of the teller at the same time, as different members portray different aspects of the teller's self. This allows the teller to see her different "selves" laid out in the playing space: her parental, child, adult, false, persecutory, desiring, phantasmatic selves and more. For example, in response to a story of a 30-year-old man who had difficulties moving relationships toward greater intimacy and commitment, two playing members entered the playing space: one of them portrayed the "avoidant self," while the other portrayed the "proactive self," who seeks to enter a deep, committed relationship. The simultaneous presence of two self-representations in the playing space embodies the elaboration and expansion of the self – the examination and discovery of its various elements and their interrelations and the creative exploration of the space in which each role exists as an aspect of the self.

In the theatrical response of the third sub-group reflecting Sonya's story, a playing member entered the playing space as the cashier lady. She kept repeating the words "I'm hungry," oscillating between anger and helpless-ness. She moved irritably around the playing space, frantically looking for something to eat. She grabbed the various cloths and ravenously gobbled them down, spreading the cloths across her face and then clutching them as they slid and spilled from her hands. She wanted to eat everything; she was constantly hungry and unsatisfied. This character gradually became a representation of the teller's nightmare about her own ravenous parts. At some point, another character entered, timidly asking, "Excuse me, is there anything to eat?" This character was the "introvert" teller. The cashier-turned-ravenous-teller looked at the timid figure of the introvert teller with rage and loathing and said, "Yes! You!" She slowly advanced toward the introvert teller, who stepped back in horror, trying to mollify the figure of the ravenous teller by saying, "just one cookie!" "This is the last one!"

This version revolved around uncontrollable, animal desire and the anx-iety about its possessiveness and voraciousness. This desire is experienced as capable of taking over one's entire inner stage. In this version, Sonya's awkwardness and introversion are presented as a result of her terror of her own animal desire and the possibility that it will take over.

The ability to hold together, within a single theatrical image, a variety of (sometimes opposing, sometimes ambivalent) voices, roles and self-states enables the reinforcement of a sense of integration and the establishment of an experience of one's self which is both complex and coherent. This al-lows the person to develop the ability to recognize their self as comprising a range of different aspects, augmenting their ability to contain and accept more diverse aspects of their self, even those which might once have been rejected or defined as "not-me." This process bolsters one's sense of self-acceptance and self-worth.

New endings, corrections and future images

Theatrical response offers an infinite space of possibilities for further developing a story's narrative. After the response is over, the conductor can put the teller back in control and suggest that they construct a different image of the future, with the help of the other members. The teller can ask the members to make a certain element of the image they created more pro-nounced or accurate or even ask them to create a new image entirely or explore different possibilities by creating corrective theatrical images. For example, a 40-year-old man shares his great difficulty with his boss, who keeps "giving him a hard time." The teller, who is unable to share the way he feels with his boss, asks to see a scene where he does answer back, telling his boss everything he wanted to be able to say to him in real life.

Another aspect of the corrective potential introduced by dramatic reality is the ability to acknowledge the missing parts of the story, the gaps that leave the story open and unfinished for the teller – the missing pieces of the puzzle. Dramatic reality allows for the expansion of reality and for adding layers and dimensions that did not exist in the story or in the teller's original experience. Therapeutic intervention in Psychotherapeutic Playback Theater seeks to help the teller acknowledge such missing pieces, those aspects that they would have liked to complete or correct. As a part of this process, members can create for the teller a fantasy image based on the teller's own wishes or on what the other members dare to dream for them. Reliving an experience and correcting its inherent lacks is one of the most significant therapeutic factors in group therapy (Yalom & Leszcz, 1995).

The theatrical response presented by the fourth sub-group in response to Sonya's story set up an imaginary scene where Sonya, her boyfriend and the cashier all met at a café to celebrate Sonya's birthday. At some point, the waiter brought a cake with candles on top and Sonya made a wish – "I want for us to stay together forever" – and then blew out the candles. This version stressed Sonya's search for relatedness in the story, her wish to connect to the cashier, the baker and the boyfriend. Still, whenever she expressed the wish for connection, she ended up frustrated and alone. This version posits intimacy as the wish through which correction takes place and the cookies as a comforting substitute for relationships.

Novel compositions

The theatrical response allows for the repositioning and reorganization of psychic elements and their theatrical representations in the playing space. Playing space positions vary in terms of upstage and downstage and different heights; the proximity of the characters or the distance between them are a meaningful expression of the composition or, in a way, the syntax of psychic material. By moving, changing places and creating new compositions in the playing space one can create new syntax for the corresponding representations in the teller's inner world, thus reorganizing various psychic materials.

The theatrical response presented by the fifth sub-group in response to Sonya's story created a dramatic resonance in which two members entered the playing space: one played "the big mother" and the other played "the little daughter." The "big mother" stood on a chair wrapped in a large cloth, a kind of cloak that covered her and the chair all the way down to the floor. The "little daughter" sat on a little chair facing her. The "little daughter" asked the "big mother" for comfort and support and the "big mother" offered her a magical cookie that would help her grow, just like the one in *Alice in Wonderland*. But the cookie had a side effect: she made the "little daughter" bigger but then shrank her right back down.

In this example, the use of playing space composition was a key element in the reflection, which exposed the psychic and archetypal structures underpinning the story. The search for confirmation by an external figure – represented in the story by the cashier and Sonya's boyfriend – entails the promise of growth, but eventually leaves Sonya small and alone. This is one way in which playing space compositions can serve to express a statement that has great psychic significance.

In general, the group-creative process of Psychotherapeutic Playback Theater fundamentally applies surrealist principles by the very fact that each member alternates between telling, performing and being a spectator in a situation where they can be present, witness and spectator their own life story. The opportunity to share a story and then watch it being performed as a tangible piece of theater by other group members is an experience that has a creative, world-making and reality-transcending element, which promotes development. The teller offers their story and a part of the passive audience rises to act. This, in itself, is a practically surreal situation. Members are not always certain whether they are performing the teller's story or their own; they find themselves within the narrative of another person, playing personal roles and intimate situations from their own lives. This process involves a blending of identities and a blurring of boundaries between members as a vital factor of the creative process. Yet another element that entails a surreal experience is the sharing circle that follows the theatrical response. At this stage, members turn from spectators and performers into tellers, sharing similar experiences to that of the teller. Taken together, these elements create a surreal experience that involves the dreamlike elements of condensation and role exchange.

In conclusion, this chapter depicted the inspiration that Psychotherapeutic Playback Theater has drawn from the surrealist movement in art, through the creation of tangible images that unfold the world of the mind through theatrical representations. Elements such as dramatic roles, movement between times and places, the expression of internal voices, exchanging roles, the use of images, movement and metaphors are all manifestations of the language of the dream, which is the language of the psyche, thus enabling a profound encounter with the inner world.

Warm-up exercises for developing the surrealist idiom

This final section presents three warm-up exercises that can help develop the ability to express metaphoric and surreal dream language when improvising in Psychotherapeutic Playback Theater.

Evolving an image through movement

The conductor asks the members to move about the room. The conductor occasionally calls out a certain image, inviting the members to move in ways that correspond to how this image makes them feel. For example, "imagine that you are water in a glass and see what type of movement this image inspires in you." In this manner, the members experience a set of different images: water in a pot, a fire being lit, water heating up, boiling, pasta, sea, jellyfish, shark, clouds, rain, field, tomatoes, a single tomato... This exercise allows one to experience an internal encounter with a given image, its attendant qualities and the various ways in which it can be expressed through movement. The fast and free transition between images and their kinetic expression highlights action and the creative flexibility it introduces.

Image dialogue through movement

This exercise is often done in groups of three. One member tells a story and the other two listen and think of an image inspired by this story. Each of the two listeners then presents their image through movement. Next, the two listeners meet and engage in a movement dialogue between their respective images. Finally, all three briefly share their experiences throughout this process.

Working through movement brings member in contact with an unknown idiom, raising the potential for a more creative encounter with the story's materials. In addition, movement allows for greater room for interpretation, so that the teller can more easily project material from their inner world onto the theatrical piece. The more abstract the image, the more interpretations one can offer.

If your Story was my dream[1]

The group is divided into groups of threes: one member tells a story and the other two listen. Then, one of the two listeners begins their reflection with the words, "if your story was my dream," and then tells a kind of dream that they have made up in response to the story. While they are recounting this made-up dream, the third member plays out what they are saying through movement. The two listeners then switch roles, so that the third member now shares a made-up dream and the second one plays it out through movement. Finally, all three members briefly share their experience of the process.

This exercise allows group members to practice their capacity for dream-thinking – for thinking in imaginative, associative and even idiosyncratic ways. It demonstrates the immense value of this type of thinking for gaining deeper insight, via unconscious channels, both into the story and into the interpersonal relations between members.

Note

1 This exercise is based on a Playback theater pattern developed in Russia, called "If That Was My Dream."

Afterword – from a house to a village on the bridge

Ronen Kowalsky, Nir Raz, Shoshi Keisari

The process of creating a layered theory that is both grounded in the academic fields of psychoanalysis, theater, art history and philosophy and based on spontaneous, lived experience is inherently laden with contradictions. Our many years in the field and the extensive experience accumulated while developing the ideas presented in this book have led us to the understanding that contradictions eventually become paradoxes, which are able to hold seemingly incommensurable aspects as parts of one whole. The process of conducting psychotherapy through *Playback Theater* works in a similar manner: it embraces both group-psychoanalytic therapy and performative theatrical improvisation, producing profound resonances through both mirroring and imaginative expansion. The opportunity for growth embedded in Psychotherapeutic Playback Theater draws on the gap between the individual and the community and that between flexible, creative flow and stable, static structure. All these components lead to the paradoxical moment when the individual suddenly recognizes themselves in new ways – as if looking in the mirror for the very first time. In these paradoxical moments, the different aspects of the individual's experience are present side by side, complementing each other in a deeply transformative manner.

One of the words that come up again and again when people are asked to describe their experience in Psychotherapeutic Playback Theater groups is "magic" – "I don't know how, but it felt like magic." Members talk about moments of being deeply touched. This is because the process facilitates a creative-collective experience that combines feelings of belonging, acceptance, being seen and feeling liberated: growth-promoting feelings are concretely inherent in it.

Throughout our years of practicing and exploring this field, we have often tried to explain this "magic." In supervision sessions, in workshops and in the classes given at the Institute for Psychotherapeutic Playback Theater, we have explored this magic and observed it from various perspectives. Through therapeutic processes and encounters with clients, students and supervisors, through case presentations and meetings with different groups and demographics, we have learned a great deal. Experiences began accumulating, leading to insights which, in turn, led to overarching concepts. All these have had a significant impact, informing and reshaping our technique. This process continued, taking shape and forming its own vocabulary throughout the writing of this book. In fact, we used a kind of reverse engineering to observe the process of Psychotherapeutic Playback Theater as a psychoanalytic group therapy process. In so doing, we witnessed the physical manifestation of psychoanalytic – the exchange of psychic material, internalization, projective identification, mirroring, containment, self-states, transitional space and more – as these were given concrete theatrical representation in the process of Psychotherapeutic Playback Theater.

While writing, we discovered a spool of thread – the same spool which vanishes and reappears before those observing the "fort-da" game (Freud, 1920, pp. 14–15; see introduction) – that holds a jumble of different layers, internal contradictions and paradoxes. This book presents our attempt to unspool this intricate thread so that it could guide the step of conductors who choose to embrace this emerging field of therapy, helping them capture, define and understand the meaning of those magical moments.

In one of our favorite interventions in Psychotherapeutic Playback Theater, "And Beyond," we ask playing members to extend their expression, in theatrical, movement-based and metaphoric means, beyond the end point of the story, as told by the teller. This intervention highlights the fact that the point at which we choose to end our story is informed by our subjective interpretation of the events – even though the story, much like life itself, goes on. What, then, is the "beyond" of this book?

The book opens a door to a vast space, most of which is still uncharted. There is ample room for studies that will explore the many variations of Psychotherapeutic Playback Theater and its potential adaptations to the needs of different client populations. Such research is needed in order to validate this emerging field and secure its place in the eyes of mental health professionals, welfare workers, educators and other decision-makers. Additional avenues of research include the potential combination of Psychotherapeutic Playback Theater with other therapeutic approaches – psychodrama, other forms of drama therapy, art therapy, movement therapy, bibliotherapy, group analysis and cognitive-behavioral group therapy. Moreover, we have yet to explore to interface between psychic space and social-collective space in terms, for example, of how Psychotherapeutic Playback Theater groups help empower communities and allow for better coping with social and political conflict. On the community level, we are curious to explore the conduction of performance-oriented Playback Theater as a large-group intervention. Finally, while this book focused on the level of group therapy, we believe it is possible to develop and practice Psychotherapeutic Playback Theater with individuals as well. We hope this book serves as a point of departure and a foundation for these and other processes, through which we can continue to build more and more houses on the bridge until, one day, we will have an entire village.

Bibliography

Ahlin, G., (2019). The group-analytic group matrix concept. *Group Analytic Society Contexts,* issue 84. https://groupanalyticsociety.co.uk/contexts/issue-84/ga-concepts-and-methods/the-group-analytic-group-matrix-concept/

Ali, A., Wolfert, S., Lam, I. & Rahman, T. (2018). Intersecting modes of aesthetic distance and mimetic induction in therapeutic process: Examining a drama-based treatment for military-related traumatic stress. *Drama Therapy Review, 4*(2), 153–165.

Apel, W. & Daniel, R. (2013) [1960]. *The Harvard brief dictionary of music.* Cambridge, MA: Harvard U.P.

Aristotle (2008). *The Poetics* (transl. S. H. Buchner). *Gutenberg Project* http://www.gutenberg.org/files/1974/1974-h/1974-h.htm. Accessed 20 September 2020.

Aristotle. (2013). *Poetics.* Oxford: Oxford University Press.

Artaud, A. (1938/1994). *The theater and its double.* London: Grove Press.

Ayalon, O. (1993). Death in literature and literature as therapy. In R. Malkinson, S. Rubin & A. Witztum (Eds.), *Loss and bereavement in Israeli society* (pp. 155–177). Jerusalem: Ministry of Defense (pp. 87–103). [Hebrew].

Barak, A. (2013). Playback theatre and narrative therapy: Introducing a new model. *Dramatherapy, 35*(2), 108–119.

Barclay, C. R. (1994). Composing protoselves through improvisation. In U. Neisser & R. Fivush (Eds.), *The remembering self: Construction and accuracy in the self-narrative* (pp. 55–77). New York: Cambridge University Press.

Beck, A. P. (1981). A study of group phase development and emergent leadership. *Group, 5*(4), 48–54.

Bernieri, F. J. & Rosenthal, R. (1991). Interpersonal coordination: Behavior matching and interactional synchrony. In R. S. Feldman & B. Rime (Eds.), *Fundamentals of nonverbal behavior* (pp. 401–432). Cambridge: Cambridge University Press.

Bion, W. R. (1961). *Experiences in groups and other papers.* London: Tavistock.

Bion, W. R. (1962). *Learning from experience.* London: Tavistock.

Bion, W. R. (1963). *Elements of psycho-analysis.* London: Heinemann.

Bion, W. R. (1967). Notes on memory and desire. *The Psychoanalytic Forum, 2*(3), 272–280.

Bion, W. R. (1967/1984). *Second thoughts.* London: Routledge.

Bion, W. R. (1970). *Attention and interpretation.* London: Maresfild.

Bion, W. R. (1978). *A seminar held in Paris.* Retrieved from http://www.psychoanalysis.org.uk/bion78.htm

Bion, W. R. (1984). *Transformations*. London: Karnac Books.

Bion, W. R. (1992). *Cogitations*. London: Karnac Books.

Blatner, A. (2000). *Foundations of psychodrama: History, theory and practice* (4th edition). New York: Springer.

Blatner, A. & Blatner, A. (1988). *Foundations of psychodrama: History, theory and practice*. New York: Springer.

Biran, H. (2015a). Point of view: Group therapy as a space for experience versus individual therapy as a space for reflection. In T. Eini-Lehman & R. Shai (Eds.), *A group story: Group therapists and facilitators write about their journey with groups* (pp. 58–76). Even Yehuda: Amatzia Books. [Hebrew]

Biran, H. (2015b). *The courage of simplicity: Essential ideas in the work of W. R. Bion*. London: Rutledge.

Boal, A. (1995). *The rainbow of desire: The Boal method of theatre and therapy*. London: Routledge.

Borges, J. L. (1949/1998). The Aleph. In A. Hurley (Ed.), *Collected fictions*. New York: Penguin Classics.

Breton, A. (1969). Manifestoes of surrealism. Ann Arbor: University of Michigan Press (Original worked published 1924).

Bromberg, P. M. (1993). Shadow and substance: A relational perspective on clinical process. *Psychoanalytic Psychology, 10,* 147–168.

Bruner, J. S. (1990). *Acts of meaning*. Cambridge, MA: Harvard University Press.

Bruner, J. S. (2004). Life as narrative. *Social Research, 71*(3), 691–710.

Caines, R. & Heble, A. (2015). *The improvisation studies reader: Spontaneous acts*. London: Routledge.

Carroll, L. (2011). *Alice in wonderland*. New York: Harper Collins.

Casson, J. (2016). Shamanism theatre and dramatherapy. In S. Jennings & C. Holmwood (Eds.), *Routledge international handbook of dramatherapy* (pp. 125–134). Abingdon: Routledge.

Chesner, A. (2002). Playback theatre and group communication. In A. Chesner & H. Herb (Eds.), *Creative advances in group work* (pp. 40–66). Philadelphia, PA: Jessica.

Cole, D. (1975). *The theatrical event: A mythos, a vocabulary, a perspective*. Middleton, CT: Wesleyan University Press.

Dauber, H. (1999). Tracing the songlines: Searching for the roots of playback theatre. In J. Fox & H. Dauber (Eds.), *Gathering voices: Essays on playback theatre* (pp. 67–76). New York: Tusitala.

Duggan, M. & Grainger, R. (1997). *Imagination, identification and catharsis in theatre and therapy*. London: Jessica Kingsley.

Eliade, M. (1972). *Shamanism: Archaic techniques of ecstasy*. Princeton: Princeton U.P.

Emunah, R. (1994). *Drama therapy process, technique and performance*. New York: Brunner/Mazel.

Emunah, R. (2020). *Acting for real: Drama therapy process, technique, and performance* (2nd ed.). New York & London: Routledge.

Fanés, F. & Fanés, F. (2007). *Salvador Dali: The construction of the image, 1925–1930*. New Haven, CT: Yale University Press.

Fairbairn, W. R. D. (1954). *An object-relations theory of the personality*. Oxford: Basic Books.

Ferenczi, S. (1933/1949). Confusion of the tongues between the adults and the child (the language of tenderness and of passion). *International Journal of Psycho-Analysis, 30*, 225–230.

Floodgate, S. (2006). *The shamanic actor: Playback theatre acting as shamanism.* Retrieved from http://www.playbacktheatre.org/wpcontent/uploads/2010/04/Floodgate_Shamanism.pdf

Fontana, D. (1997). *Teach yourself to dream.* San Francisco, CA: Chronicle Books.

Foulkes, S. H. (1964). *Therapeutic group analysis.* London: Allen and Unwin.

Foulkes, S. H. (1990). *Selected papers of S. H. Foulkes: Psychoanalysis and group analysis.* London: Karnac.

Foulkes, S. H. & Anthony, E. J. (1965). *Group psychotherapy: The psychoanalytic approach.* London: Karnac Books.

Fox, H. (2007). Playback theatre: Inciting dialogue and building community through personal story. *The Drama Review, 51*(4), 89–105.

Fox, J. (1994). *Acts of service: Spontaneity, commitment, tradition in the nonscripted theatre.* New York: Tusitala.

Fox, J. (1999). A ritual for our time. In J. Fox & H. Dauber (Eds.), *Gathering voices: Essays in playback theatre* (pp. 9–16). New Paltz, NY: Tusitala.

Fox, J. (2007). *Playback Theatre compared to psychodrama and theatre of the oppressed.* Retrieved from http://www.playbackschool.org/pt_compared_psy_and_to.htm

Freud, S. (1900). The interpretation of dreams. *The Standard edition of the complete psychological works of Sigmund Freud* (Vol. IV, pp. 1–338). London: Hogarth.

Freud, S. (1912/1990). Recommendations for physicians on the psycho-analytic method of treatment. In R. Langs (Ed.), *Classics in psychoanalytic technique* (pp. 391–396). Lanham, MD: Rowman & Littlefield.

Freud, S. (1917). *A general introduction to psychoanalysis.* London: Andesite Press.

Freud, S. (1920). *Beyond the pleasure principle* (standard ed., Vol. XVIII, pp. 7–64). London: Hogarth Press.

Friedman, R. (2002). Dreamtelling as a request for containment in group therapy. In K. Neri, M. Pines & R. Friedman (Eds.), *Dreams in group psychotherapy: Theory and technique* (pp. 46–67). London: Jessica Kingsley.

Friedman, R. (2017). The group analysis of the Akeda: The worst and the best feelings in the matrix. In R. Friedman & Y. Doron (Eds.), *Group analysis in the land of milk and honey* (pp. 61–74). London: Rutledge.

Gergen, K. J. (1991). *The saturated self: Dilemmas of identity in modern life.* New York: Basic Books.

Gergen, K. J. & Gergen, M. M. (1988). Narrative and the self as relationship. *Advances in Experimental Social Psychology, 21*, 17–56.

Gersie, A. & King, N. (1990). *Storymaking in education and therapy.* London: Jessica Kingsley Publishers.

Greimas, A. (1991). Debates with Paul Ricoeur. In M. Valdes (Ed.), *Reflection and imagination: A Ricoeur reader.* London: Harvester Wheatsheaf.

Grotowski, J. (1968). *Towards a poor theatre.* New York: Simon & Schuster.

Hammer, M. (1972/2015). *The theory and practice of psychotherapy with specific disorders.* Retrieved from https://www.israpsych.org/books/wp-content/uploads/2015/12/theory-and-practice-of-psychotherapy-with-specific-disorders.pdf

Harrison, J. (2009). Any road. In *Let it roll: Songs by George Harrison.* London: Apple Records.

Hodermarska, M., Benjamin, P. & Omens, S. (2016). The play as client: An experiment in autobiographical therapeutic theatre. In S. Pendzik, R. Emunah & D. Johnson (Eds.), *The self in performance* (pp. 255–266). New York: Palgrave Macmillan.

Hopper, E. (2003a). *The social unconscious: Selected papers.* London: Jessica Kingsley Publishers.

Hopper, E. (2003b). *Traumatic experience in the unconscious life of groups: The fourth basic assumption: Incohesion: Aggregation/massification or (ba) I/A/M.* London: Jessica Kingsley Publishers.

Hopper, E. (2018). The development of the concept of the tripartite matrix: A response to 'Four modalities of the experience of others on groups' by Victor Schermer. *Group Analysis, 51*(2), 197–206.

Hopper, E. (2020). The tripartite matrix, the basic assumption of incohesion and scapegoating in foulkesian group analysis: Clinical and empirical illustrations, including terrorism and terrorists. *Forum, 8,* Online.

Huizinga, J. (1949/2002). *Homo Ludens: A study of the play-element in culture.* London: Routeldge.

International Playback Theatre Network (IPTN). (2018). *The community voice of playback theatre.* Retrieved from www.iptn.info

Jennings, S. (1998). *Introduction to dramatherapy: Theatre and healing.* London: Jessica Kingsley.

Johnson, D. R. (1996). The drama therapist "in role." In S. Jennings, (Ed.), *Dramatherapy theory and practice, Vol. 2* (pp.112–136). London: Routledge.

Johnson, D. R. (2009). Developmental transformations: Toward the body as presence. In D. Johnson & R. Emunah (Eds.), *Current approaches in drama therapy* (pp. 89–116). Springfield, IL: Charles C. Thomas.

Jung, C. G. (1960). *On the nature of the psyche.* Princeton: Princeton University Press.

Jung, C. G. (1964). *Man and his symbols.* London: Aldus Books.

Jung, C. G. (1916/2003). *Psychology of the unconscious.* New York: Dover Publications.

Kabat-Zinn, J. (1994). *Wherever you go, there you are: Mindfulness meditation in everyday life.* New York: Hyperion.

Kant, I. (1998). *Critique of pure reason* (Tr. P. Guyer and A. W. Wood). Cambridge: Cambridge University Press.

Keisari, S. (2021). Expanding older adults' role repertoire through drama therapy: An integrative model. *Frontiers in Psychology, 12,* 635975.

Keisari, S., Raz, N. & Kowalsky, R. (2018). MacKenzie on stage: A group development through psychotherapeutic playback theatre. *Mikbatz, 23*(1): 73–90. [Hebrew].

Keisari, S., Yaniv, D., Palgi, Y. & Gesser-Edelsburg, A. (2018). Conducting playback theatre with older adults: A therapist's perspective. *The Arts in Psychotherapy, 60,* 72–81.

Keisari, S., Gesser-Edelsburg, A., Yaniv, D. & Palgi, Y. (2020). Playback theatre in adult day centers: A creative group intervention for community-dwelling older adults. *PloS One, 15*(10), e0239812.

Keisari, S., Palgi, Y., Yaniv, D. & Gesser-Edelsburg, A. (2020). Participation in life-review playback theater enhances mental health of community-dwelling older adults: A randomized controlled trial. *Psychology of Aesthetics, Creativity, and the Arts.* doi:10.1037%2Faca0000354

Kernberg, O. F. (1995). *Object relations theory and clinical psychoanalysis.* New York: Jason Aronson.

Kim, H. & Mastnak, W. (2015). Creative Pansori: A new Korean approach in music therapy. *Voices, 15*(3). doi:10.15845/voices.v16i1.816

Klein, M. (1946). Notes on some schizoid mechanisms. *International Journal of Psycho-Analysis, 27,* 99–110.

Klein, M. (1975). *The writings of Melanie Klein.* London: Hogarth Press and the Institute of Psycho-Analysis.

Kohut, H. (1959). Introspection, empathy, and psychoanalysis an examination of the relationship between mode of observation and theory. *Journal of the American Psychoanalytic Association, 7*(3), 459–483.

Kohut, H. (1971). *The analysis of the self.* London: Hogath Press.

Kohut, H. (1977). *The restoration of the self.* Chicago: University of Chicago Press.

Kohut, H. (1984). *How does analysis cure?* Chicago: University of Chicago Press.

Kohut, H. & Wolf, E. (1978). The disorders of the self and their treatment: An outline. *The International Journal of Psychoanalysis, 59,* 413–425.

Kossak, M. (2015). *Attunement in expressive arts therapy: Toward an understanding of embodied empathy.* Springfield, IL: Charles C. Thomas.

Kowalsky, R. (2014). *The hall of mirrors on stage.* The Institute of Psychotherapeutic Playback Theater First Annual Conference, Netanya, Israel.

Kowalsky, R., Keisari, S. & Raz, N. (2019). Hall of mirrors on stage: An Introduction to Psychotherapeutic Playback Theatre. *The Arts in Psychotherapy, 66,* 1–7.

Kristeva, J. (1986). *The Kristeva reader.* Oxford: Blackwell.

Kulka, R. (2013). Psyche or soul in psychoanalysis: Towards the conceptualization of play as a psychoanalytic transcendental selfobject. In E. Perroni, J. Green & P. Gandolfi (Eds.), *Play: Psychoanalytic perspectives, survival and human development* (pp. 47–61). London: Routledge.

Lacan, J. (1984). *Escritos, 1.* México: Siglo XX.

Lacan, J. (2001). *Ecrits: A selection.* Oxon: Routledge.

Lahad, M. (2006). *Fantastic reality: Creative supervision in therapy.* Tivon: Nord. [Hebrew].

Landy, R. (1993). *Persona and performance: The meaning of role in drama, therapy and everyday life.* New York: Guilford.

Landy, R. (1996). Drama therapy and distancing: Reflections on theory and clinical application. *The Arts in Psychotherapy, 23*(5), 367–373.

Landy, R. (2000). Role theory and the role method of dramatherapy. In P. Lewis & D. R. Johnson (Eds.), *Current approaches in drama therapy* (pp. 65–89). Springfield, IL: Charles C. Thomas.

Landy, R. J. (2006). The future of drama therapy. *The Arts in Psychotherapy, 33*(2), 135–142.

Landy, R. J., Luck, B., Conner, E. & McMullian, S. (2003). Role profiles: A drama therapy assessment instrument. *The Arts in Psychotherapy, 30*(3), 151–161.

Langer, S. (1953). *Feeling and form.* New York: Charles Scribner's Sons.

Levinas, E. (1969). *Totality and infinity: An essay on exteriority.* Paris: Duquesne.

Levinas, E. (1987). *Time and the other.* Pittsburgh: Duquesne University Press.

Lubrani-Rolnik, N. (2009). *Life in a Story: Playback theatre and the art of improvisation*. Tel Aviv: HaKibbutz HaMeuhad. [Hebrew].

Lurie, L. (2013). Play as a world of magic and drama: Winnicott's ideas about play in their application to children's psychotherapy. In E. Perroni, J. Green & P. Gandolfi (Eds.), *Play: Psychoanalytic perspectives, survival and human development* (pp. 33–46). London: Routledge.

Machado, A. (2003). *There is no road* (Tr. M.G. Berg and D. Maloney). Buffalo, NY: White Pine Press.

MacKenzie, K. R. (1990). *Introduction to time-limited group psychotherapy*. Washington, DC: American Psychiatric Pub.

MacKenzie, K. R. & Livesley, W. J. (1983). A developmental model for brief group therapy. In R. R. Dies & K. R. MacKenzie (Eds.), *Advances in group psychotherapy: Integrating research and practice* (pp. 101–116). New York: International Universities Press.

Mahler, M. (1967). On human symbiosis and the vicissitudes of individuation. *Journal of the American Psychoanalytic Association, 15*(4), 740–763.

McAdams, D. P. (2001). The psychology of life stories. *Review of General Psychology, 5*(2), 100–122.

Moran, G. S. & Alon, U. (2011). Playback theatre and recovery in mental health: Preliminary evidence. *The Arts in Psychotherapy, 38*(5), 318–324.

Moreno, J. J. (2006). The music therapist: Creative arts therapist and contemporary shaman. In D. Campbell (Ed.), *Music physician for times to come* (pp. 167–185). Wheaton, IL: Quest Books.

Moreno, J. L. (1946/1985). *Psychodrama, first volume* (4th ed.). New York: Beacon House.

Moreno, J. L. (1961). The role concept, a bridge between psychiatry and sociology. *American Journal of Psychiatry, 118*, 518–523.

Moreno, J. L. (1965). Therapeutic vehicles and the concept of surplus reality. *Group Psychotherapy and Psychodrama, 18*, 211–216.

Moreno, J. L. (1987). In J. Fox (Ed.), *The essential Moreno: Writings on psychodrama, group method, and spontaneity by J. L. Moreno, M.D.* (pp. 57–78). New York: Springer.

Moreno, J. L. & Moreno, Z. T. (1969). Psychiatry of the twentieth century: Function of the universalia – Time, space, reality and cosmos. *Psychodrama: Action Therapy and Principles of Practice, 3*, 11–23.

Moreno, J.J. (2016). The music therapist: Creative arts therapist and contemporary shaman. *International Journal of Psychotherapy, Counseling and Psychiatry*. doi:10.35996/1234/2/arttherapyshaman. Accessed 18 September 2020.

Moreno, Z. T., Blomkvist, L. D. & Rutzel, T. (2013). *Psychodrama, surplus reality and the art of healing*. New York: Routledge.

Murray, K., Epston, D. & White, M. (1992). A proposal for re-authoring therapy: Rose's revision of her life and a commentary. In S. McNamee & K. Gergen's (Eds.), *Therapy as social construction* (pp. 96–115). London: Sage.

Nadler, A. (1999). *The history of psychology: A reader*. Tel Aviv: Tel Aviv University. [Hebrew].

Neumann, E. (1989). *The origin and history of consciousness*. London: Karnac.

Ogden, T. H. (1979). On projective identification. *International Journal of Psycho-Analysis, 60*, 357–373.

Ogden, T. H. (1992). *The primitive edge of experience.* New York: Jason Aaronson.

Ogden, T. H. (1994). *Object of analysis.* New York: Jason Aronson.

Ogden, T. H. (2003). On not being able to dream. *The International Journal of Psychoanalysis, 84*(1), 17–30.

Ogden, T. H. (2004). On holding and containing, being and dreaming. *International Journal of Psychoanalysis, 85,* 1349–1364.

Osterweil, Z. (1995). *Open solutions: The psychological treatment of children.* Jerusalem: Schoken. [Hebrew].

Pallaro, P. (Ed.) (1999). *Authentic movement: A collection of essays by Mary Starks Whitehose, Janet Adler and Joan Chodorow.* London: Jessica Kingsley.

Peled, E. (2005). *Psychoanalysis and Buddhism: About the capacity to know.* Tel Aviv: Resling. [Hebrew].

Pendzik, S. (1988). Drama therapy as a form of modern shamanism. *Journal of Transpersonal Psychology, 20,* 81–92.

Pendzik, S. (2004). Uberlegungen zu Schamanismus und Praktiken der Dramatherapie: Das Beispiel von Dona Joaquina. In R. Krey & V. Merz (Eds.), *Feministische Reflexionen* (pp. 142–163). St Gallen: BoD.

Pendzik, S. (2006). On dramatic reality and its therapeutic function in drama therapy. *The Arts in Psychotherapy, 33*(4), 271–280.

Pendzik, S. (2008). Dramatic resonances: A technique of intervention in drama therapy, supervision, and training. *The Arts in Psychotherapy, 35*(3), 217–223.

Pendzik, S. (2013). The 6-key model and the assessment of the aesthetic dimension in dramatherapy. *Dramatherapy, 35*(2), 90–98.

Pendzik, S. (2016). Dramatherapy and the feminist tradition. In S. Jennings & C. Holmwood (Eds.), *The international handbook of dramatherapy* (pp. 306–316). London: Routledge.

Pendzik, S. (2018). Drama therapy and the invisible realm. *The Drama Therapy Review, 4*(2), 182–197.

Pendzik, S., Emunah, R. & Johnson, D. R. (2017). *Self in performance.* New York: Palgrave Macmillan.

Pines, M. (1984). Reflections on mirroring. *International Review of Psycho-Analysis, 11,* 27–42.

Pines, M. (1985). Mirroring and child development. *Psychoanalytic Inquiry, 5*(2), 211–231.

Pitruzzella, S. (2004). *Introduction to drama therapy: Person and threshold.* Hove and New York: Bruner-Routledge.

Pitruzzella, S. (2017). *Drama, creativity and intersubjectivity.* Abingdon: Routledge.

Polkinghorne, D. (1988). *Narrative knowing and the human sciences.* Albany: State University of New York Press.

Ray, P. & Pendzik, S. (2021). Autobiographical therapeutic performance as a means of improving executive functioning in traumatized adults. *Frontiers in Psychology, 12.* doi:10.3389/fpsyg.2021.599914

Ricks, L., Kitchens, S., Goodrich, T. & Hancock, E. (2014). My story: The use of narrative therapy in individual and group counseling. *Journal of Creativity in Mental Health, 9*(1), 99–110.

Riessman, C. K. (2008). *Narrative methods for the human sciences.* Los Angeles, CA: Sage.

Ryvko, J. (2005). A dream in a psychodrama group as a group voice. *Nefesh, Quarterly for Psychology, Therapy, Emotional Care and Creative Education, 19–20*, 111–125. [Hebrew].

Ryvko, J. (2018). *First act then know: Experience and studying psychodrama and group work*. Azor: Tzameret Books. [Hebrew].

Rogers, C. R. (1986). Reflection of feelings and transference. *Person-Centered Review, 1*, 375–377.

Rosenthal, G. (1993). Reconstruction of life stories: Principles of selection in generating stories for narrative biographical interviews. In R. Josselson & A. Lieblich (Eds.), *The narrative study of lives* (pp. 59–91). Newbury Park, CA: Sage.

Rowe, N. (2007). *Playing the other: Dramatizing personal narratives in playback theatre*. London: Jessica Kingsley.

Sajnani, N., (2012). The implicated witness: Towards a relational aesthetic in dramatherapy. *Dramatherapy, 34*(1), 6–21.

Sajnani, N. & Johnson, D. R. (2011). Opening up playback theatre: Perspectives from theatre of the oppressed and developmental transformations. Retrieved from http://www.playbacktheatre.org/wp-content/uploads/2011/03/Opening-Up-Playback-Theatre-.pdf. Accessed 1 August 2017.

Salas, J. (1993). *Improvising real life: Personal story in playback theatre*. New York: Tusitala Publishing.

Salas, J. (2007). *Do my story, sing my song: Music therapy and playback theatre with troubled children*. New Paltz, NY: Tusitala Publishing.

Salas, J. (2009). Playback theatre: A frame of healing. In D. R. Johnson & R. Emunah (Eds.), *Current approaches in drama therapy* (pp. 445–460). Springfield, IL: Charles C. Thomas.

Sartre, J. P. (1949). *No exit and three other plays*. New York: Vintage Books.

Sartre, J. P. (2000). *Nausea*. London: Penguin.

Schafer, R. (1983). *The analytic attitude*. New York: Basic Books.

Schechner, R. (2005). *Performance theory*. London and New York: Routledge.

Schlapobersky, J. (2016). *From the couch to the circle: Group-analytic psychotherapy in practice*. London: Routledge.

Shakespeare, W. (2009). *As you like it*. Cambridge: Cambridge University Press.

Shapiro, S. (2009). The integration of mindfulness and psychology. *Journal of Clinical Psychology, 65*(6), 555–560.

Shtadler, R. (2017). *Stories in treatment: Healing stories as "Third" in the psychotherapy*. Haifa: Pardes. [Hebrew].

Smigelsky, M. A. & Neimeyer, R. A. (2018). Performative retelling: Healing community stories of loss through Playback Theater. *Death Studies, 42*(1), 26–34.

Snow, S. (2009). Ritual/theatre/therapy. In D. R. Johnson & R. Emunah (Eds.), *Current approaches to drama therapy* (pp. 117–144). Springfield, IL: Charles C. Thomas.

Stafford, W. (1994). *The darkness around us is deep: Selected poems*. New York: Harper Perennial.

Stern, D. (1983). The early development of schemas of self, other and 'self' with other. In J. D. Lichtenberg & S. Kaplan (Eds.), *Reflections on self-psychology* (pp. 49–84). Hillsdale, NJ: The Analytic Press.

Stern, D. (2002) [1977]. *The first relationship: Infant and mother*. London: Harvard U.P.

Stueber, K. R. (2012). Varieties of empathy, neuroscience and the narrativist challenge to the contemporary theory of mind debate. *Emotion Review, 4*(1), 55–63.

Sletvold, J. (2015). Embodied empathy in psychotherapy: Demonstrated in supervision. *Body, Movement and Dance in Psychotherapy, 10*(2), 82–93.

Todar, M. & Weinberg, H. (2006). The group through the looking glass. *Mikbatz – The Israel Journal of Group Psychotherapy, 11*(1), 35–54. [Hebrew].

Turner, V. (1982). *From ritual to theatre: The human seriousness of play.* New York: PAJ Publications.

Tuckman, B. W. (1965). Developmental sequence in small groups. *Psychological Bulletin, 63*(6), 384–399.

Walcot, P. (1976). *Greek drama in its theatrical and social context.* Cardiff: University of Wales Press.

White, M. (2000). *Reflections on narrative practice: Essays and interviews.* Adelaide: Dulwich Centre.

White, M. (2007). *Maps of narrative therapy.* New York: W. W. Norton & Company.

White, M. & Epston, D. (1990). *Narrative means to therapeutic ends.* New York: W. W. Norton & Company.

Winnicott, D. W. (1949). Mind and its relation to the psyche-soma. In D. W. Winnicott (Ed.), *Through paediatrics to psycho-analysis* (pp. 243–254). London: The Hogarth Press, 1975.

Winnicott, D. W. (1965). Ego distortions in terms of true and false self. In M. Masud & R. Khan (Eds.), *The maturational process and the facilitating environment* (pp. 140–152). New York: International Universities Press.

Winnicott, D. W. (1971). *Playing and reality.* New York: Basic Books.

Wood, S. M. (2018). Transforming families using performance: Witnessing performed lived experience. *Drama Therapy Review, 4*(1), pp. 23–37.

Yalom, I. D. & Leszcz, M. (1995). *The theory and practice of group psychotherapy.* New York: Basic Books.

Yotis, L., Theocharopoulos, C., Fragiadaki, C. & Begioglou, D. (2017). Using playback theater to address the stigma of mental disorders. *The Arts in Psychotherapy, 55*, 80–84.

Zarrilli, P. (2006). Oral, ritual, and shamanic performance. In G. J. Williams (Ed.), *Theatre histories: An introduction* (2nd ed.) (pp. 15–39). London: Routledge.

Zinkin, L. (1983). Malignant mirroring. *Group Analysis, 16*(2), 113–126.

Zinkin, L. (1993). Exchange as a therapeutic factor in group analysis. In D. Brown & L. Zinkin (Eds.), *The psyche and the social world: Developments in group analytic theory* (pp. 99–117). London: Routledge.

Zaporah, R. (2021). Action theatre home page. *Action Theatre.* Available at http://actiontheatre.com

Zoran, G. (2009). *Beyond mimesis: Text and textual arts in Aristotelian thought.* Tel Aviv: Tel Aviv University. [Hebrew].

Index

For Product Safety Concerns and Information please contact our EU
representative GPSR@taylorandfrancis.com Taylor & Francis Verlag GmbH,
Kaufingerstraße 24, 80331 München, Germany

Printed and bound by CPI Group (UK) Ltd, Croydon, CR0 4YY
08/06/2025
01897006-0010